THE COMPLETE RENAL DIET COOKBOOK

THE
COMPLETE
RENAL DIET
COOKBOOK

Stage-by-Stage Nutritional Guidelines,
Meal Plans, and Recipes

Emily Campbell, RD, CDE, MScFN

ROCKRIDGE
PRESS

For general information on our other products and services or to obtain technical support, please contact our Customer Care Department within the United States at (866) 744-2665, or outside the United States at (510) 253-0500.

Rockridge Press publishes its books in a variety of electronic and print formats. Some content that appears in print may not be available in electronic books, and vice versa.

TRADEMARKS: Rockridge Press and the Rockridge Press logo are trademarks or registered trademarks of Callisto Media Inc. and/or its affiliates, in the United States and other countries, and may not be used without written permission. All other trademarks are the property of their respective owners. Rockridge Press is not associated with any product or vendor mentioned in this book.

Interior and Cover Designer: Amanda Kirk

Art Producer: Megan Baggott

Editor: Marjorie DeWitt

Production Editor: Mia Moran

Production Manager: Martin Worthington

Cover photography © 2021 Elysa Weitala, food styling by Victoria Woollard; Hélène Dujardin, 2; Annie Martin, 26; Eric Fenot/PhotoCuisine/StockFood USA, 42; Darren Muir, 47; Katie Neudert/StockFood USA, 60; Elysa Weitala, 69; Eising Studio/Gräfe & Unzer Verlag/StockFood USA, 77; The Picture Pantry/StockFood USA, 78, 94; Cameron Whitman/Stocksy United, 112; Pierre Louis Viel/PhotoCuisine/StockFood USA, 130; Brent Hofacker/Shutterstock, 144

Author photo courtesy of Amanda Lee / Simplee Creatives

ISBN: Print 978-1-64876-544-5 | eBook 978-1-64876-545-2

R0

To my patients and colleagues
who inspire me to develop delicious
recipes that help make nutrition
easier for those living with
kidney disease.

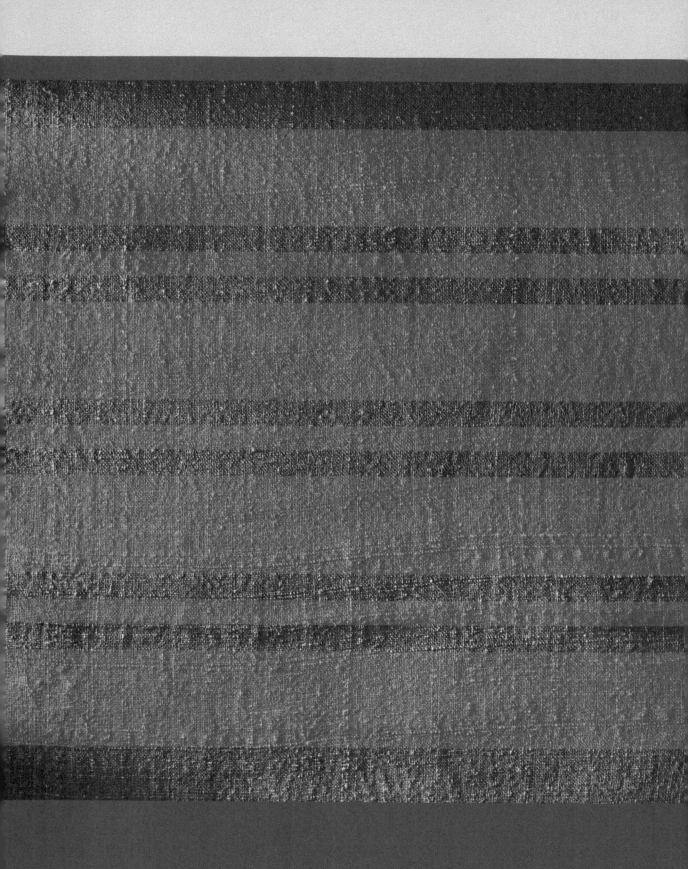

Contents

Introduction

Chronic Kidney Disease (CKD) is a condition that occurs when your kidneys become damaged and do not work as well as they should. According to the Centers for Disease Control and Prevention, someone with CKD experiences a decline in kidney function and is unable to filter wastes as well as someone with healthy kidneys. Specifically, the kidneys are unable to filter the blood effectively, causing waste products (such as urea, uric acid, and creatinine) to build up in the blood. The term "chronic" indicates that this damage has occurred over a long period of time. While CKD is not reversible, the progression of the disease, or the damage, can be delayed. Kidney damage that leads to CKD can be due to other diseases like diabetes or high blood pressure, or from genetic or autoimmune disorders. The National Kidney Foundation estimates that one in seven adults in the United States have CKD. This is important to know so that you realize you are not alone in this journey. CKD happens, but it is not a death sentence. CKD can be managed, and kidney function can be preserved and stabilized for months or years.

Nutrition plays an important role in preventing and delaying the effects of CKD. With so much information available at their fingertips, many individuals feel overwhelmed when they learn they have kidney disease. They aren't sure where to start, and navigating nutrition strategies at each stage of CKD can be confusing. Without speaking with a registered dietitian, trying to decipher protein, sodium, potassium, and phosphorus requirements (while likely managing other health problems like diabetes and high blood pressure), can get quite complicated. For example, there is a fine line between too little and too much protein for CKD stages

1 to 4. Too little can put you at risk of malnutrition, and too much makes your kidneys work harder. Dietary recommendations can change quickly, even between blood work tests, so it's no wonder many people feel frustrated with nutrition for CKD.

As a registered dietitian and certified diabetes educator with many years of experience working in this area of nutrition, I have seen the impact nutrition can have on individuals with CKD. I have helped my clients understand health recommendations, delay progression of their CKD, and live life to the fullest. I take pride in helping my clients preserve kidney function and delay the need to start dialysis. Additionally, I have family members who live with CKD, so I know firsthand how stressful mealtimes and special occasions can be. This professional and personal experience has helped me better understand the nutrition needs and wants of those with CKD.

About This Book

You probably purchased this book because you or someone you know has CKD. This book is here to help you learn more about the foods that can help or harm kidney function at every stage. Each of the 95 recipes in this cookbook provides valuable nutritional information and the critical nutrients you should pay attention to: protein, sodium, potassium, and phosphorus. Knowing this information will help you understand which recipes are most appropriate for you. The goal of this book is to support you on this lifelong journey and to maintain your health while helping you build your knowledge of a kidney-friendly diet that you can put into action. The contents of this book should not be taken as medical advice and are not a substitute or replacement for the medical advice provided to you by your doctor or dietitian.

Your CKD Journey

ACCORDING TO THE NATIONAL INSTITUTE OF DIABETES and Digestive and Kidney Diseases (NIDDK), nutrition strategies can help maintain or preserve kidney function, assist in managing associated health problems (such as diabetes, high blood pressure, or high cholesterol), and provide overall help in maintaining weight in order to improve your quality of life. Understanding kidney function is important and highly recommended so that you are well informed for making decisions on this journey.

This section covers the basics of a renal diet, portion control and calorie intake, tips for a balanced diet, and several meal plans to set you up for success. A kidney diet can be both nutritious and delicious, so let's show you how you can have both!

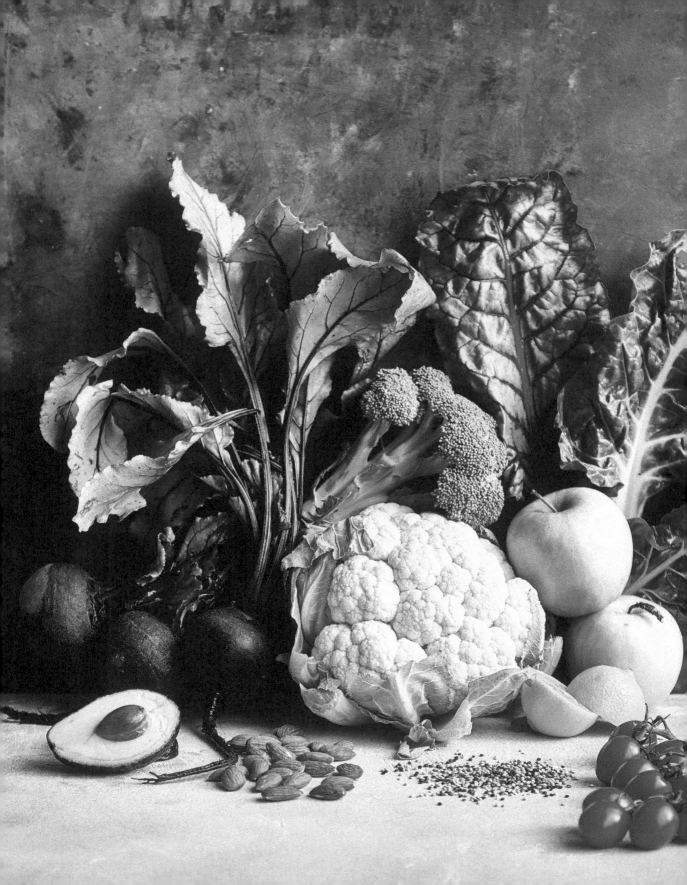

CHAPTER 1

ALL ABOUT THE RENAL DIET

The renal diet is often viewed as difficult to follow because of the number of nutrients you need to consider, but this does not need to be the case. These first two chapters will support you on your CKD journey by explaining what is happening in your body, showing you easy meals to prepare, answering protein consumption questions, and explaining the best meals to consume to delay progression of kidney disease.

Treating Chronic Kidney Disease

CKD is a progressive disease, meaning that it doesn't happen overnight but over time, typically three months or longer. The kidneys filter waste from the blood and remove excess fluid from the body. They also play a role in regulating blood pressure, keeping bones healthy, and assisting with red blood cell production. When the kidneys aren't working properly, they don't filter the blood as needed. As outlined by Dr. Michael Zemaitis in his book *Uremia*, when the kidneys are damaged and there is a decrease in function, waste products called uremia begin to build up in the blood.

The NIDDK states that more than 37 million Americans have CKD; however, many don't even know they have it because symptoms don't appear until later stages. The five stages of CKD are measured by the Estimated Glomerular Filtration Rate (eGFR), a percentage value that indicates the level of kidney function. The lower the eGFR, the lower the kidney function. As kidney function declines, waste products in the blood begin to accumulate, and other symptoms appear. These symptoms include loss of appetite, fatigue or tiredness, swelling (edema) due to fluid retention in hands or feet, bad breath or a metallic taste in the mouth, shortness of breath, decreased mental sharpness or difficulty concentrating, urinating less frequently, changes in urine color (may be foamy, dark orange, brown, or tea-color and condensed), sleep problems, muscle cramps or restless legs, and persistent itching. This is all because of the accumulation of waste products in the body.

WHAT TO ASK YOUR HEALTH-CARE TEAM

Medical appointments can be stressful or overwhelming, so taking steps to alleviate this stress is important. One of the best methods to help yourself is to take a lead role in your health care, because it can bring comfort and understanding that you'll need in order to make the right decisions for you.

Going to appointments with your questions written down will help remove some of the stress, allowing you to listen to your health-care team more closely because you won't be focused on trying to remember what else to ask. While this book provides a guide for moving forward, it is important that you discuss your individual needs with your kidney health-care team. Here is a list of questions to consider.

1. How many calories do I need?
2. Do I need to limit how much protein I eat? If so, how many grams of protein should I eat?
3. What does a balanced meal include?
4. Is my potassium level too high or low?
5. Should I restrict my phosphorus intake?
6. How much sodium (salt) should I consume?
7. How many ounces of fluid are right for me?
8. Do I need a nutritional supplement?
9. Should I take vitamins?
10. What nutrition strategies can help delay CKD progression?

Renal Diet 101

Managing CKD requires lifestyle adjustments, including diet changes. With the right diet choices, the kidneys will have less waste to filter, and kidney function can be preserved. As CKD progresses, individuals may lose their appetite or experience taste changes, which may lower their motivation to eat. For this reason, maintaining nutritional status and getting enough calories, while limiting protein and sodium, is vital.

As CKD progresses, nutrition needs change. It is important to always discuss individual needs with a kidney health-care team. To assist, this book includes dietary guidelines and meal plans for individuals with CKD stages 1 to 3, stage 4, and stage 5 (dialysis).

To begin, let's look at the critical nutrients and their impact on the body:

- *Potassium:* plays an important role with heart function. Too much or too little potassium can be dangerous. Foods with more than 200mg of potassium per ½-cup serving are considered high-potassium foods. Some packaged foods may have potassium additives. Reading food labels can help you identify these foods and choose alternatives.

- *Phosphorus:* keeps bones and teeth strong. With CKD, phosphorus can build up in the body, causing weak bones and hardened blood vessels. There are two sources of phosphorus: natural phosphorus and phosphorus additives. Natural phosphorus comes from foods like meat, dairy, and nuts; phosphorus additives are commonly found in processed foods. Reading food labels can help you identify sources of phosphorus additives.

- *Protein:* used to build muscle and fight infections. Too much protein can cause waste products to build up in the blood, making it hard for the kidneys to remove the waste.

- *Sodium:* too much sodium (salt) can lead to high blood pressure (hypertension) and swelling (edema) because the kidneys can't rid the body of the excess fluid. Sodium is a mineral found in foods as well as table salt. Most individuals consume more than the recommended intake for sodium in their diet.

- *Carbohydrates:* provide the body with an energy source. Some foods provide both soluble and insoluble fiber. Fiber is important for managing cholesterol and blood glucose (sugar) levels and keeping bowels regular. Choose whole grains (e.g., whole-grain bread, brown rice) at meals as often as possible, as these are sources of insoluble fiber. Constipation may be common for individuals with kidney problems, especially when a fluid restriction is an issue. Including whole grains and high-fiber foods for as long as possible (because these foods may also be a source of potassium) can help manage constipation.

- *Fats:* Saturated fats found in red meat, poultry, whole-fat dairy, and butter and trans fats often found in processed or packaged foods should be avoided as these can lead to high cholesterol. Choose foods with high amounts of unsaturated fat for heart health. This includes nuts (e.g., almonds and walnuts), seeds (e.g., pumpkin and sesame), and olive or canola oil. Food sources of omega-3 fatty acids such as fatty fish (e.g., salmon), nuts/seeds, and canola oil can help reduce cardiovascular events associated with CKD.

- *Fluids:* as kidney function declines, excessive fluid intake can be dangerous as it may lead to swelling because the kidneys can't rid the body of the fluid. Limit fluids only if advised by your health-care team.

- *Vitamins and minerals:* necessary for general health and body functions. Don't hesitate to ask your health-care team if a supplement is needed.

The chance of developing CKD increases with the onset of other diseases, such as diabetes, high blood pressure, heart disease, or a family history of kidney disease such as polycystic kidney disease (PKD) or immune diseases such as lupus or IgA nephropathy. NIDDK states that with the increase in age, the risk of developing CKD also increases, especially for those over 60 years, who are at the highest risk.

While there is no cure for CKD, the progression can be slowed through the help of a health-care team and by making positive changes to diet and lifestyle. The five stages of CKD are as follows:

Stage 1: Slight kidney damage with normal or increased filtration (GFR>90 mL/min)

Stage 2: Mild decrease in kidney function (GFR = 60 to 89 mL/min)

Stage 3: Moderate decrease in kidney function (GFR = 30 to 59 mL/min)

Stage 4: Severe disease in kidney function (GFR = 15 to 29 mL/min)

Stage 5: Kidney failure/end-stage CKD (GFR<15 mL/min)

The following sections provide an overview of the nutrition guidelines for each stage of CKD. Following that, there is a section on portion control and calorie intake. At the end of the book, you will find a food list with nutritional information for common foods.

■ Stages 1 to 3

In stages 1 to 3 nutrition changes focus on reducing the work of the kidneys through protein and sodium restrictions. These changes can help preserve kidney function longer.

POTASSIUM

Restriction is necessary when lab values exceed 5.0mmol/L because too much potassium could cause an irregular heartbeat. Potassium restrictions are not common in stages 1 to 3. However, if needed, limit potassium to 2000mg per day by choosing low-potassium vegetables and fruit such as apples, clementines, pineapple, arugula, bell peppers, cauliflower, and cabbage, to name a few.

PHOSPHORUS

It is important to avoid phosphorus additives completely because too much phosphorus can weaken bones and teeth. Read food labels to check for added phosphorus by looking for "phos" in the ingredient list. If lab values exceed 1.45mmol/L, limiting phosphorus intake to 1000mg per day is important. Avoid high-phosphorus foods such as cola, organ meats, and processed foods.

PROTEIN

Following a low-protein diet (0.6 to 0.8 grams per kilogram of body weight for individuals with diabetes, or 0.55 to 0.6 grams per kilogram for those without diabetes) can protect the kidneys by reducing the load they filter. Spacing protein throughout the day with three meals will also help lessen the work of the kidneys. As often as possible, choose plant-based proteins, such as tofu, legumes or beans, nuts or nut butter, and seeds.

SODIUM

Limiting sodium intake to 2300mg per day can help minimize swelling and excessive filtering for the kidneys. Reading food labels for low-sodium products and cooking with herbs and spices instead of salt can help meet this restriction.

CARBOHYDRATES

Aim for 20 to 30 grams of fiber a day by choosing high-fiber foods like whole grains (e.g., bread, rice, pasta).

FAT

Aim for a total fat intake of 25 percent to 35 percent of calories, and saturated-fat intake of less than 7 percent of calories. Choose low-fat dairy products, lean cuts of meat, and cook with plant-sterol-enriched margarine instead of butter to help reduce saturated-fat intake.

FLUIDS

A fluid restriction may not be necessary. Maintaining hydration is important, because this can help preserve kidney function. Aim for 1.5 to 2 liters of fluid per day, unless a doctor has recommended a different value because of a heart condition or swelling.

VITAMINS

A vitamin or mineral supplement is likely not necessary, unless otherwise instructed by a kidney team. Following a balanced kidney diet can help supply all the necessary nutrients.

SUMMARY

- Potassium restrictions are individualized. A low-potassium diet is 2000mg potassium per day.
- Restrict phosphorus intake to no more than 1000mg per day if your phosphorus is high; avoid foods with added phosphorus.
- Ensure your protein intake is appropriate for you (see page 15).
- Limit sodium to 2300mg per day by choosing fresh and unprocessed foods and flavoring foods with herbs and spices.

■ Stage 4

As kidney disease progresses and kidney function declines, further nutritional changes may be necessary to help manage the side effects of CKD. Individuals with stage 4 CKD may begin to require potassium and phosphorus restrictions. Preserving kidney function through protein and sodium restrictions continues with this stage. Many also experience weight loss due to a lack of appetite at this stage, so nutrition strategies to manage weight are important.

POTASSIUM

Potassium requirements may need to be adjusted to keep your blood values at target levels. If your potassium level is high (above 5.0mmol/L), a low-potassium diet may be recommended; if it's low (less than 3.5mmol/L), a high-potassium diet may be recommended. A low-potassium diet aims for 2000mg of potassium per day and includes foods such as blueberries, raspberries, grapes, cucumber, eggplant, and string beans. A high-potassium diet aims for 3500mg potassium per day and includes foods such as avocados, tomatoes, oranges, mangos, quinoa, nuts, and seeds.

PHOSPHORUS

Too much phosphorus can cause weak bones and teeth as well as lead to vein and artery hardening. If phosphorus values rise above 1.45mmol/L, a phosphorus restriction is recommended. Aim for less than 1000mg phosphorus per day by choosing low-phosphorus foods such as couscous, barley, oatmeal, lemonade, and non-cola beverages. Avoid added phosphorus by reading food labels and looking for "phos" in the ingredient list.

PROTEIN

Meeting protein needs for muscle and immune-system strength is important. The key is not to exceed the nutritional need. Continue to follow a low-protein diet (0.6 to 0.8 grams per kilogram of body weight for individuals with diabetes, or 0.55 to 0.6 grams per kilogram for those without diabetes) and aim for 50 percent from animal proteins. Half of the time, include plant-based proteins, such as legumes or beans, tofu, and nuts, as these are easier for the kidneys to filter. Note, however, that these may be high in potassium.

CARBOHYDRATES

Aim for 20 to 30 grams of fiber per day by choosing high-fiber foods such as whole grains (e.g., bread, rice, pasta). Carbohydrate foods can be great sources of calories if your appetite is low and weight loss occurs. Also try to eat two cups of fresh, frozen, or canned (no salt or sugar) vegetables or fruit per meal.

FAT

Aim for a total fat intake of 25 percent to 35 percent of calories, and saturated-fat intake of less than 7 percent of calories. Choose low-fat dairy products and lean cuts of meat and cook with plant-sterol-enriched margarine instead of butter to help reduce saturated-fat intake. Add heart-healthy calories such as nuts, seeds, olive oil, and margarine to foods if weight loss occurs.

FLUIDS

Maintaining hydration is important because this can help preserve kidney function. Aim for 1.5L to 2L of fluids per day unless a doctor has recommended a different value because of a heart condition or swelling.

SUMMARY

- Maintain weight and muscle mass by achieving your calorie needs through snacks or adding heart-healthy calories to foods.
- Target 2000mg of potassium per day if you are on a low-potassium diet, or 3500mg on a high-potassium diet.
- Limit protein to reduce the workload of your kidneys and choose plant-based proteins as often as possible.
- Limit phosphorus to 1000mg per day if your phosphorus is high. Continue to avoid phosphorus additives.
- Continue to limit sodium intake to 2300mg per day through label reading and cooking at home.

Stage 5

While on dialysis, nutrition recommendations for potassium and phosphorus will depend on how well dialysis is working. With the start of dialysis, your appetite may improve as the blood is filtered and cleaned, which can help decrease side effects.

POTASSIUM

A potassium restriction may be necessary depending on your residual kidney function, dialysis clearance, dialysis type (hemodialysis or peritoneal dialysis), and overall potassium intake. Aim for 3000mg potassium unless a restriction is needed. Individuals on peritoneal dialysis may need more potassium.

PHOSPHORUS

When the kidneys are not filtering, phosphorus can build up quickly, causing hardened blood vessels and weak bones or teeth. Phosphorus control can help prevent mortality in CKD patients and should be maintained at less than 1.78mmol/L. Limit phosphorus to 800mg to 1000mg per day by choosing fresh and unprocessed foods, cooking at home, choosing nondairy alternatives, and avoiding colas, chocolate, and organ meats. Continue to avoid added phosphorus by reading food labels for "phos" in the ingredient list of cereals, bread, or packaged products. Many individuals on dialysis may also require medications often referred to as "phosphorus binders" to help remove phosphorus from the blood. It is important to take these medications as prescribed with your food to help prevent excess phosphorus from building up in the blood.

PROTEIN

Protein needs to increase when on dialysis, because you lose protein during treatment. This helps preserve muscle mass. Aim for 1.0g to 1.2g per kilogram of body weight per day for individuals on dialysis. Protein needs can be met with a plant-based protein; however, some individuals may prefer animal proteins to meet their needs.

SODIUM

Limiting sodium intake to 2300mg per day can help minimize swelling and excessive filtering requirements of the kidneys. Reading food labels for low-sodium products and cooking with herbs and spices instead of salt can help meet this restriction.

CARBOHYDRATES

Aim for 20g to 30g of fiber a day by choosing high-fiber foods such as whole grains (e.g., bread, rice, pasta). Aim for two cups of vegetables or fruit per meal.

FAT

Aim for a total fat intake of 25 percent to 35 percent of calories, and saturated-fat intake of less than 7 percent of calories. Choose low-fat dairy products and lean cuts of meat and cook with plant-sterol-enriched margarine instead of butter to help reduce saturated-fat intake.

FLUIDS

With kidney failure, urine output will decrease, so any fluids you take in may accumulate in your body between dialysis sessions. For those on hemodialysis, limit fluids to urine output plus 1L. Individuals of peritoneal dialysis may not require a fluid restriction as their dialysis occurs more frequently. Fluids include water, coffee, tea, juice, soup, ice cream, and yogurt. Basically, anything that becomes liquid at room temperature.

VITAMINS

A kidney-safe multivitamin may be recommended by your health-care team to help prevent or treat micronutrient deficiencies.

SUMMARY

- Aim for 3000mg potassium; adjust depending on lab values.
- Limit phosphorus to 800 to 1000mg per day; continue to avoid added phosphorus.
- Protein needs are higher; aim for 1.0 to 1.2g/kg.
- Limit fluid to 1L plus urine output, on hemodialysis.
- Continue to limit sodium intake to 2300mg per day.

Stage-by-Stage Nutritional Needs

This table summarizes the nutritional need for each stage of CKD.

CKD STAGE	1 TO 3	4	5
Potassium	Individualized.	Individualized.	Aim for 3000mg/day.
Phosphorus	Avoid added phosphorus.	Limit to 1000mg/day. Avoid added phosphorus.	Limit to 800 to 1000mg/day. Avoid added phosphorus.
Sodium	Limit to 2300mg/day.	Limit to 2300mg/day.	Limit to 2300mg/day.
Protein	0.6 to 0.8g/kg body weight per day for individuals with diabetes, 0.55 to 0.6g/kg body weight for no diabetes	0.6 to 0.8g/kg body weight per day for individuals with diabetes, 0.55 to 0.6g/kg body weight for no diabetes	1.0 to 1.2g/kg body weight per day
Fluids	Individualized.	Individualized.	Individuals on hemodialysis should limit fluids to what their urine output is per day plus 1L. Individuals on peritoneal dialysis may not require a fluid restriction because dialysis occurs more frequently.
For Diabetes	Aim for 30 to 45g of carbohydrates per meal and 15g of carbohydrates per snack. Read food labels for high-fiber foods with 4g of fiber per serving. Avoid added sugars.	Aim for 30 to 45g of carbohydrates per meal and 15g of carbohydrates per snack. Choose high-fiber foods. Avoid added sugars.	Aim for 30 to 45g of carbohydrates per meal and 15g of carbohydrates per snack. Choose high-fiber foods. Avoid added sugars.
For Hyper-tension	Aim for three meals per day and half a plate of vegetables or fruit at each meal. Cook with fresh herbs and spices. Read food labels for low-sodium products.		
Additional Notes	None.	Adjust potassium levels depending on blood work. Low-potassium diets should be 2000mg/day; high-potassium diets should be 3500mg/day.	Adjust potassium levels depending on blood work. Low potassium is 2000mg/day; high potassium is 3500mg/day

Portion Control and Caloric Intake

Portion control and enjoying a variety of kidney-friendly foods is important in managing CKD. It's known that people struggle to understand proper portion sizes, but success can be achieved if you think of it as balancing food group portions on a plate. Aim for one-half plate of vegetables, one-fourth plate of protein, and one-fourth plate of carbohydrates. Have three meals per day, no more than four to six hours apart. This time line helps spread the protein load your kidneys process throughout the day, thus minimizing their work while also meeting macronutrient and micronutrient needs. The half a plate of vegetables with each meal provides adequate fiber, manages blood glucose and cholesterol levels, and helps with having regular bowel movements. Incorporate fruit by choosing fruit as a snack. Practice protein portion control by limiting it to a quarter of the plate. This will help preserve kidney function and prevent waste products from building up. Choose foods prepared with less salt by buying fresh foods and cooking from scratch. Limit processed or prepared foods—use fresh herbs and spices to season food—in order to help control blood pressure. Make water your beverage of choice.

Consuming enough calories is important for preventing weight loss and malnutrition. Aim for 25 to 35 calories per kilogram of body weight per day to meet energy needs. Many individuals may experience weight loss when following a kidney-friendly diet because of calorie and nutrient restrictions, or changes in taste, which can lead to a decreased appetite. If maintaining body weight becomes a challenge, work with a registered dietitian for a personalized plan.

To calculate calorie needs, multiply your weight in kilograms by 25 and 35 calories per kilogram. To calculate weight in kilograms, divide your weight in pounds by 2.2. For example, an individual who weighs 165 pounds (or 75 kilograms) requires 1875 to 2250 calories per day (75kg × 25 calories/kg = 1875 calories, and 75kg × 30 calories/kg = 2250 calories).

ADJUSTING FOR ASSOCIATED CONDITIONS

According to Davita Kidney Care, diabetes, high blood pressure, and heart disease are commonly found with CKD. Together, they are referred to as a "silent partnership" because they are often overlooked until they reach advanced stages and their symptoms become noticeable. CKD can develop from uncontrolled diabetes and/or uncontrolled high blood pressure. Many individuals with end-stage CKD do not die of kidney failure itself, but from heart disease. Keeping blood glucose and blood pressure levels under control helps slow the progression of kidney disease. The recipes in this book will help with all of these conditions, resulting in a healthier life.

The following are tips that can be made to the recipes to help accommodate diabetes, high blood pressure, and heart disease when meal planning:

Diabetes

- Limit the addition of added sugars (including honey, sugar, or maple syrup) in recipes.
- Choose bulgur or parboiled rice instead of white rice as these are lower in glycemic index, meaning they do not cause the blood glucose to rise as quickly or as high.
- Make water your beverage of choice.

Blood Pressure

- Choose no added salt (sometimes shortened to "NAS" or "NSA") canned products.
- Read food labels for low-sodium options. Aim for 600mg per serving per meal and 200mg per snack or condiment.
- Incorporate fresh or dried herbs for flavoring instead of salt.
- Cook at home from scratch.

Heart Disease

- Choose heart-healthy oils, such as olive oil, or a plant-sterol-enriched margarine instead of unsalted butter or lard.
- Incorporate plant-based or vegetarian meals more often, swap ground beef with lentils.
- Aim for three servings of heart-healthy fish per week, such as salmon, shrimp, tuna, or tilapia.

Your Kidney-Friendly Kitchen

Having the right equipment readily available can make your life easier when cooking. These basic cooking utensils will help speed up meal prep when preparing these recipes.

Equipment and Tools

Most of these items are common and in most kitchens, but let's be prepared:

Blender: Used to mix or blend foods, this kitchen staple is great for making smoothies and sauces.

Food processor: Used to chop, mix, or puree foods, this is a great tool for making dips, chopping hard foods, and pureeing ingredients together.

Grill or panini press: The ultimate tool for making sandwiches, these toast the bread and warm the sandwich fillings, without having to flip the sandwich.

Medium cast-iron skillet: Great for cooking and keeping foods warm for longer and includes additional health benefits for people with anemia. As explained by P. D. Geerligs in his article about anemia, cast-iron skillets can help with anemia because they are a source of iron for the diet. Anemia can be prevalent with CKD patients because the kidneys produce hormones that make red blood cells. When kidney function declines, individuals with CKD are at risk of anemia because this hormone production is low. Outside sources of iron are important.

Pastry cutter: A small tool used for blending flour and butter together to make pastries. A fork can also be used for this purpose.

Pantry Essentials

Keeping a small stock of the following pantry items can make recipe preparation easy, especially when making meals in a hurry. These basic and versatile items are used frequently and have a long shelf life. This pantry list includes 30 of the most common items used over and over again in the recipes in this book. Build your pantry over time by choosing a few recipes in the book to begin with.

- All-purpose flour
- Applesauce, unsweetened
- Baking soda
- Chia seeds, whole
- Chili powder
- Cinnamon, ground
- Cream of tartar
- Cumin, ground
- Garlic, powder and fresh
- Ginger, powder and fresh
- Honey

- Old-fashioned rolled oats
- Olive oil
- Onion powder
- Paprika
- Parsley, dried
- Pasta, lasagna
- Pasta, orzo
- Pasta, spaghetti
- Peanut butter, unsalted
- Red pepper flakes, dried
- Red wine vinegar

- Reduced-sodium soy sauce
- Rice, parboiled
- Rice vinegar
- Rosemary, dried
- Sesame oil
- Thyme, dried
- Vanilla extract
- White vinegar

SMART SHOPPING

Grocery shopping is a significant household expense. Shopping smart with the following tips can help make grocery shopping more convenient and affordable.

MORE CONVENIENT:

Opt for prepared ingredients at the grocery store. Choose prewashed and chopped vegetables and fruit. This can save time in the kitchen and encourage higher consumption of both.

Make a list. Shop efficiently by creating a list by grocery store sections (produce, dairy, staples, and necessities).

Get your groceries delivered. This can save you time and ensure that extra or unnecessary items don't end up in the cart.

MORE AFFORDABLE:

Purchase staple items in bulk. Purchasing long-life staple items like rice, pasta, or cereal in bulk can help save money over time. Look for the longest expiration date when buying.

Read store flyers. Use the flyers to help inspire meal plans for the week and save money. Look for in-store promotions.

Don't shop hungry. Going shopping hungry will often lead to impulse purchases.

Price match. Compare prices between stores and see if stores will match lower prices elsewhere.

Tips for Dietary Success

Being on a restrictive diet can be challenging, but there are tools to make it work. The following prescriptive tips will help.

Meal Planning and Preparation

Practice meal planning by using the meal plan and shopping lists in this book. Over time, and as comfort and knowledge of the kidney diet grows, use the plate method to plan meals, and adapt recipes for protein, sodium, potassium, and phosphorus based on need.

There are many ways to meal prep, and choosing a method that will work for you will help set you up for success.

Make-ahead meals: Prepare full meals and refrigerate for use later. For example, if you skip breakfast each day, try preparing breakfast ahead of time so you can grab it and go in the morning.

Batch cooking: Make a large batch of a recipe and freeze portions to be eaten later.

Ready-to-cook ingredients: Prepare ingredients for specific meals ahead of time. For example, if you are having pasta a few different days, cook the pasta for the week ahead of time.

Helpful Tracking Tools

Keeping track of food intake can provide insight into what your body has to work with. Two tools to check out that could help are the calorie tracker from Cronometer .com and the food analyzer from the Davita Kidney Care website (Davita.com).

Eating Out

Before dining out, review the menu online or in person, and look for low-sodium options. Ask for modifications to be made to your meal, such as no salt and condiments on the side, as these can be high sources of sodium. Try splitting a meal with a friend or taking the rest home for later. Request smaller portions of certain items, like protein, if needed. Choose meals you can customize.

Cravings

Adjusting to a new lifestyle can be difficult when unhealthy cravings pop up. It can create a guilty feeling toward certain foods. Instead of feeling deprived or guilty, try modifying the recipe or have a small portion of the craved food on special occasions.

Reading Food Labels

Reading food labels and ingredient lists can provide important information on sources of sodium, potassium, and phosphorus and will also indicate if additives like potassium and phosphorus are included. Avoid foods with words beginning with "potassium" or "phos" in their ingredients, as these identify potassium and phosphorus additives. Look at the food label to determine if a food has a little or a lot of sodium. Aim for 600mg or less per serving for meals, and 200mg or less per snack or condiment.

HEALTHY LIFESTYLE CHANGES

Nutrition is only one aspect of helping manage CKD. It is also important to support your physical and mental health. The following strategies can help improve life quality and kidney disease outcomes.

Exercise daily. Physical activity is important for delaying kidney disease progression and managing diabetes and heart disease. Start with 10 minutes of exercise per day, and work up to a goal of 30 minutes or more per day. Start with low-impact options like walking, swimming, or yoga. Whenever adding something new to your health plan, speak with a health-care provider before starting.

Manage stress. When you experience stress, the physiological reactions to stress can increase blood pressure, which in turn can damage the kidneys. Set time aside time to relax and use relaxation techniques like yoga or meditation. Talking to a friend or loved one can help reduce stress and provide support. Seek out further support from a health-care provider if needed.

Get enough sleep. The kidneys help regulate your sleep-wake cycle, so getting enough sleep is important. To help increase and improve sleep, limit caffeine before bed, create a bedtime routine where bedtime is consistent each night, reduce screen time before bed, and do not use your cell phone in bed.

Avoid kidney stressors. Cigarettes, alcohol, and painkillers can cause rapid loss in kidney function. Speak to a health-care professional for strategies on how to reduce or avoid kidney stressors.

Staying Positive

With a new diagnosis of a chronic disease and adjusting to a new lifestyle, it is common to get overwhelmed or discouraged. No one is perfect, and slipups will happen. Learn from those mistakes and embrace this new lifestyle. Keep an open mind; learn, grow, and stay positive. Before you get into the nitty-gritty of the renal diet, here are tips for success:

Learn about the disease. Knowledge is power, and this power will help establish control for a healthy lifestyle and build a foundation for a positive attitude.

Take it one step at a time. Focus on one nutrient at a time. Going from zero to 100 with diet changes typically doesn't set most people up for success.

Find a reason to be grateful. Saying thank you, writing in a gratitude journal, or being grateful in other ways has been shown to increase positivity, which in turn, improves health.

Go for a walk. Walking produces positive hormones called endorphins. These hormones increase happiness and improves energy.

Talk to people. Join a support group to meet others with CKD; having support from people who understand the challenges can help with adjusting to new routines, increasing learning, and developing a growth mindset.

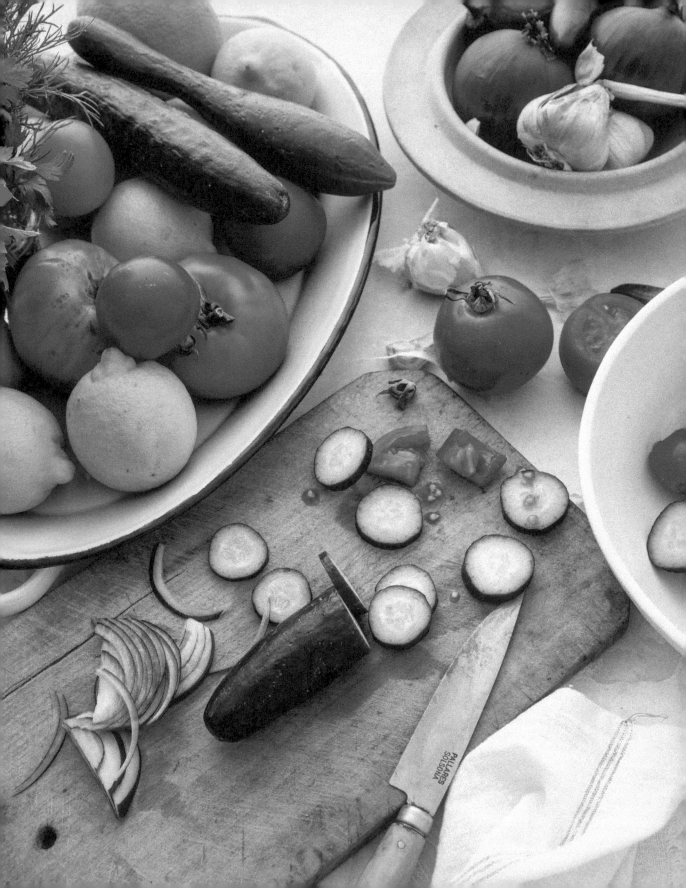

CHAPTER 2

STAGE-BY-STAGE MEAL PLANS

Planning ahead helps you get the most out of your meals, saves time in the kitchen, and keeps food costs down. Meals cooked at home tend to be lower in sodium and saturated fat, which is important when managing CKD and preventing associated conditions. Planning nutritious meals can seem daunting, stressful, or confusing, so here is the help you need. In this section you will find meal ideas to help build your confidence with healthy kidney-friendly eating.

About the Plans

Meal planning starts with making lists. You will want to note the foods you have in the house and the foods you need to pick up at the store. Keeping a running list each week of foods used will help with organization and make shopping easier and less frequent.

Keeping a list of favorite recipes, like the ones in this cookbook, can help direct your meal plans each week. Read grocery store flyers for inspiration on what foods to buy, including foods that are in season and bulk sale items. Save time by using leftovers for lunch or for another meal later in the week, or save things for later by freezing them. Aim to always include at least one serving of vegetables and/or fruit per meal for a balanced fiber-filled meal. Having the proper supplies to store foods is also important so be sure to have airtight containers with fitting lids and materials that wash and freeze well. Being organized with containers lowers stress and big messes.

The meal plans included in this cookbook are designed for one person. Each one-week meal plan is organized by kidney stage with accompanying shopping lists and time-saving tips. Also included in the meal plans are recipe staples from this cookbook; however, store-bought substitutions can be used to save time. Feel free to swap in different fruits, vegetables, or proteins in the meals to better suit your preferences. If you want to add a salad as a side item, go for it. Just be sure to add the necessary ingredients to your shopping list. While everyone's needs vary, working with a registered dietitian can help you determine the best personalized meal plan for you.

STAGES:　■1–3　■4　■5

■ Stages 1–3

WEEK 1

	MONDAY	TUESDAY	WEDNESDAY	THURSDAY	FRIDAY	SATURDAY	SUNDAY
Breakfast	Blueberry, Strawberry, and Cauliflower Smoothie (page 45)	Blueberry, Strawberry, and Cauliflower Smoothie (leftovers)	Apple Muesli (page 49)	Apple Muesli (leftovers)	Strawberry, Raspberry, and Kale Smoothie (page 44)	Strawberry, Raspberry, and Kale Smoothie (leftovers)	Blueberry Pancakes (page 46)
Lunch	Pineapple Fried Rice (page 87)	Minestrone (page 82)	Pineapple Fried Rice (leftovers)	Minestrone (leftovers)	Tofu Pad Thai (leftovers)	Chicken Stuffed Peppers (leftovers)	Pork Tenderloin Stuffed with Apples and Onions (leftovers) with Sweet and Savory Mashed Squash and Carrots (leftovers)
Dinner	Lemon-Butter Tilapia (page 98) with Garlic Double-Boiled Mashed Potatoes (page 66)	Lemon-Butter Tilapia (leftovers) with Garlic Double-Boiled Mashed Potatoes (leftovers)	Minestrone (leftovers)	Tofu Pad Thai (page 81)	Chicken Stuffed Peppers (page 119)	Pork Tenderloin Stuffed with Apples and Onions (page 118) with Sweet and Savory Mashed Squash and Carrots (page 62)	Honey, Lime, and Garlic Baked Salmon (page 102) with Tangy Garlic-Roasted Brussels Sprouts (page 63)
Snack	Honey-Vanilla Energy Balls (page 67)	Honey-Vanilla Energy Balls (leftovers)	4 ounces plain yogurt and 1 small apple	½ cup grapes and 1 ounce mozzarella cheese	½ cup pineapple and 1 ounce unsalted almonds	Honey-Vanilla Energy Balls (leftovers)	1 clementine and 1 ounce unsalted almonds

■ Stages 1–3

	WEEK 2						
	MONDAY	**TUESDAY**	**WEDNESDAY**	**THURSDAY**	**FRIDAY**	**SATURDAY**	**SUNDAY**
Breakfast	Blueberry-Lentil Muffin (page 52)	Blueberry-Lentil Muffin (leftovers)	Cherry Oatmeal (page 50)	Cherry Oatmeal (leftovers)	Apple Scone and Yogurt (page 48)	Strawberry, Raspberry, and Kale Smoothie (page 44)	Blueberry Pancakes (leftover from week 1)
Lunch	Honey, Lime, and Garlic Baked Salmon (leftover from week 1) with Tangy Garlic-Roasted Brussels Sprouts (leftovers)	Mediterranean Turkey Burgers (leftovers) and Crunchy Cauliflower Salad (leftovers)	Minestrone (leftover from week 1)	Lemon Tofu (page 80)	Lemon Tofu (leftovers)	Spicy Ginger Tilapia Soup (page 99)	Spicy Ginger Tilapia Soup (leftovers)
Dinner	Mediterranean Turkey Burgers (page 120) and Crunchy Cauliflower Salad (page 65)	Shrimp Spaghetti (page 100)	Shrimp Spaghetti (leftovers)	Chicken Cacciatore (page 116) with Garlic Double-Boiled Mashed Potatoes (leftover from week 1)	Chicken Cacciatore (leftovers) with Garlic Double-Boiled Mashed Potatoes (leftover from week 1)	Caribbean Seasoned Chicken (page 117)	Caribbean Seasoned Chicken (leftovers)
Snack	½ cup pineapple and 1 ounce unsalted almonds	Honey-Vanilla Energy Balls (leftovers)	4 ounces plain yogurt and 1 clementine	Honey-Vanilla Energy Balls (leftovers)	Honey-Vanilla Energy Balls (leftovers)	½ cup grapes and 1 ounce mozzarella cheese	4 ounces plain yogurt and strawberries

Shopping List

PRODUCE

- Apples, large (2)
- Apples, small (5)
- Bell peppers, green (5 large)
- Bell peppers, green (7 medium)
- Blueberries, fresh or frozen (5½ cups)
- Bok choy, chopped (1 cup)
- Brussels sprouts, halved (2 cups)
- Carrots (6 large)
- Cauliflower head (2 medium)
- Celery stalk (1)
- Cherries, fresh (½ cup)
- Clementines (2)
- Coleslaw mix, cabbage and carrot (3 cups)
- Garlic heads (2)
- Ginger, fresh (4 inches)
- Grapes (1 cup)
- Green beans (1 cup)
- Kale, chopped (1 cup)
- Lemon juice (4 ounces)
- Lemons (2)
- Lime juice (3 ounces)
- Limes (5)
- Onion, white (1 large)
- Onions, white (5 medium)
- Pineapple, fresh (1½ cups)
- Potatoes, white (2 medium)
- Raspberries, fresh or frozen (1 cup)
- Scallions (6)
- Snap peas (2 cups)
- Squash, spaghetti (1 small)
- Strawberries, fresh or frozen (2½ cups)

DAIRY AND EGGS

- Almond milk, unsweetened plain (1 [64-ounce] carton)
- Butter, unsalted (2 sticks)
- Cheese, part-skim mozzarella (2 ounces)
- Eggs (6 large)
- Kefir, plain (1 [32-ounce] carton)
- Sour cream (1 [8-ounce] container)
- Yogurt, plain probiotic, 2% (1 [32-ounce] container)
- Yogurt, plain Greek, 2% (1 [5-ounce] container)

MEAT AND SEAFOOD

- Chicken, ground (5 ounces)
- Chicken thighs, skinless and boneless (12 ounces)
- Pork tenderloin (1 pound)
- Salmon, fresh (8 ounces)
- Shrimp, fresh or frozen (½ pound)
- Tilapia, fresh (14 ounces)
- Turkey, ground (5 ounces)

PANTRY

- Baking soda
- Black pepper
- Broth, no-salt-added chicken (1 [32-ounce] carton)
- Broth, no-salt-added vegetable (2 [32-ounce] cartons)
- Chia seeds
- Chili powder
- Cinnamon, ground
- Cooking spray
- Cream of tartar
- Cumin, ground
- Diced tomatoes, no-salt-added (2 [14.5-ounce] cans)
- Flour, all-purpose
- Garlic powder
- Honey
- Lentils, no-salt-added (1 [14-ounce] can)
- Noodles, rice (4 ounces)
- Oats, old-fashioned rolled
- Olive oil
- Onion powder
- Paprika
- Parsley, dried
- Pasta, orzo (4 ounces)
- Pasta, spaghetti (16 ounces)
- Peanut butter
- Pineapple chunks, juice-packed (4 [8-ounce] cans)
- Red pepper flakes
- Rice, parboiled
- Rosemary, dried
- Soy sauce, reduced-sodium
- Tomato paste, low-sodium (1 [5-ounce] can)
- Vanilla extract
- Vinegar, red wine
- Vinegar, rice
- Vinegar, white

OTHER

- Almonds, unsalted
- Applesauce, unsweetened
- Buns, hamburger or brioche (4)
- Tofu, firm (14 ounces)

Prep Ahead

There are a few things you can prepare ahead to save time or simplify the process:

- Prep the rice for both the Chicken Stuffed Peppers (page 119) and Pineapple Fried Rice (page 87) recipes at the same time. Store the cooked rice in the refrigerator for use later.

- Freeze leftover Blueberry Pancakes (page 46) and warm them up for a quick weekday breakfast.

- The shopping list will prepare servings for multiple days. Keep two servings available for the meal plan, and freeze leftovers of these recipes to enjoy later: Lemon Butter Tilapia (page 98), Tofu Pad Thai (page 81), Pineapple Fried Rice (page 87), Chicken Stuffed Peppers (page 119), Pork Tenderloin Stuffed with Apples and Onions (page 118), Sweet and Savory Mashed Squash and Carrots (page 62), Honey, Lime, and Garlic Baked Salmon (page 102), and Tangy Garlic-Roasted Brussels Sprouts (page 63), Mediterranean Turkey Burgers (page 120), Shrimp Spaghetti (page 100), Spicy Ginger Tilapia Soup (page 99), Chicken Cacciatore (page 116), and Caribbean Seasoned Chicken (page 117).

- Make the Honey-Vanilla Energy Balls (page 67) and keep them in the freezer until you're ready to use them. This helps keep them fresh longer. Take them out the day before you want to eat them to let them thaw.

- Make the Minestrone (page 82), store two servings in the refrigerator for use on Tuesday and Wednesday of Week 1. Freeze the remaining two portions. Remove one portion Wednesday evening to let thaw overnight in time for Thursday's lunch. The last portion should be thawed overnight to be ready for lunch on Wednesday in Week 2. Make the Garlic Double-Boiled Mashed Potatoes (page 66) and store two servings in the freezer for use in Week 2. Thaw out overnight when ready to use.

- Prepare the Rosemary-Garlic Sauce (page 154) for the turkey burgers ahead of time to let the flavors marinate. This can be kept in the refrigerator for five days.

Stage 4

	MONDAY	TUESDAY	WEDNESDAY	THURSDAY	FRIDAY	SATURDAY	SUNDAY
Breakfast	Berry and Chia Seed Pudding (page 54)	Berry and Chia Seed Pudding (leftovers)	Cherry Oatmeal (page 50)	Cherry Oatmeal (leftovers)	Blueberry, Strawberry, and Cauliflower Smoothie (page 45)	Blueberry, Strawberry and Cauliflower Smoothie (leftovers)	Blueberry Pancakes (page 46)
Lunch	Grilled Paneer Sandwich (page 88)	Grilled Paneer Sandwich (leftovers)	Peanut-Chili Tofu with Noodles (page 90)	Peanut-Chili Tofu with Noodles (leftovers)	Spicy Panfried Tilapia (page 106) with Garlic Double-Boiled Mashed Potatoes (page 66)	Spicy Panfried Tilapia (leftovers) with Garlic Double-Boiled Mashed Potatoes (leftovers)	Spicy Salmon (page 103) with Chili Roasted Broccoli (page 73)
Dinner	Mushroom Chicken with Rosemary and Thyme (page 122) with Lemon-Garlic Green Beans (page 74)	Mushroom Chicken with Rosemary and Thyme (leftovers) with Lemon-Garlic Green Beans (leftovers)	Shrimp Fried Rice (page 101)	Shrimp Fried Rice (leftovers)	Pineapple-Glazed Chicken Thigh Stir-Fry (page 123) with Roasted Carrots and Leeks (page 70)	Pineapple-Glazed Chicken Thigh Stir-Fry (leftovers) with Roasted Carrots and Leeks (leftovers)	Chickpea Curry (page 89)
Snack	1 clementine and 1 ounce unsalted almonds	Honey-Vanilla Energy Balls (page 67)	4 ounces plain yogurt and 1 clementine	½ cup grapes and 1 ounce mozzarella cheese	Honey-Vanilla Energy Balls (leftovers)	1 small apple and 1 ounce unsalted almonds	Honey-Vanilla Energy Balls (leftovers)

Shopping List

PRODUCE

- Apple, small (1)
- Bell peppers, green (5 medium)
- Blueberries, fresh or frozen (4½ cups)
- Broccoli heads (2)
- Carrots (10 medium)
- Cauliflower florets (½ cup)
- Cherries, fresh (½ cup)
- Clementines (2)
- Garlic heads (2)
- Ginger, fresh (6 inches)
- Grapes (½ cups)
- Green beans (3 cups)
- Leeks (3)
- Lemon juice (3 ounces)
- Lime juice (1 ounce)
- Mushrooms, portobello (2)
- Mushrooms, white button (1 pint)
- Onions, red (2 small)
- Onions, white (4 medium)
- Potatoes, white (2 medium)
- Raspberries (1 cup)
- Strawberries, fresh or frozen (1½ cups)

DAIRY AND EGGS

- Almond milk, unsweetened plain (1 [64-ounce] carton)
- Butter, unsalted (1 stick)
- Cheese, mozzarella (1 ounce)
- Eggs (3 large)
- Paneer (3 ounces)
- Yogurt, plain, 2% (1 [5-ounce] container)

MEAT AND SEAFOOD

- Chicken thighs, skinless and boneless (10 ounces)
- Salmon, skin on (8 ounces)
- Shrimp, fresh or frozen (4 ounces)
- Tilapia, fresh (8 ounces)

PANTRY

- Baking soda
- Black pepper
- Chia seeds
- Chickpeas, no-salt-added (1 [15-ounce] can)
- Chili powder
- Cinnamon, ground
- Cooking spray
- Cream of tartar
- Cumin, ground
- Flour, all-purpose
- Garlic powder
- Honey
- Oats, old-fashioned rolled
- Olive oil
- Onion powder
- Oregano, dried
- Paprika
- Parsley, dried
- Pasta, spaghetti (4 ounces)
- Peanut butter, unsalted
- Pineapple chunks, juice-packed (2 [8-ounce] cans)
- Red pepper flakes
- Rice, parboiled
- Roasted red peppers (1 [12-ounce] jar)
- Rosemary, dried
- Sesame oil
- Sourdough loaf (1)
- Soy sauce, reduced-sodium
- Thyme, dried
- Tomato sauce, no-salt-added (1 [15-ounce] can)
- Vanilla extract
- Vinegar, rice
- Vinegar, white

OTHER

- Almonds, unsalted
- Tofu, firm (6 ounces)

Prep Ahead

The shopping list will prepare servings for multiple days. Keep two servings available for the meal plan, and freeze the extra portions of these recipes for another day: Peanut-Chili Tofu with Noodles (page 90), Spicy Panfried Tilapia (page 106), Garlic Double-Boiled Mashed Potatoes (page 66), Mushroom Chicken with Rosemary and Thyme (page 122), Lemon-Garlic Green Beans (page 74), Shrimp Fried Rice (page 101), Pineapple-Glazed Chicken Thigh Stir-Fry (page 123), Roasted Carrots with Leeks (page 70), Chickpea Curry (page 89), and Honey-Vanilla Energy Balls (page 67). The Spicy Salmon (page 103) and Chili Roasted Broccoli (page 73) each will only make one serving.

Stage 5

	WEEK 1						
	MONDAY	**TUESDAY**	**WEDNESDAY**	**THURSDAY**	**FRIDAY**	**SATURDAY**	**SUNDAY**
Breakfast	High-Protein Oatmeal (page 57)	High-Protein Oatmeal (leftovers)	Peach-Pineapple Protein Smoothie (page 56)	Peach-Pineapple Protein Smoothie (leftovers)	High-Protein Oatmeal (page 57)	Cream Cheese–Stuffed French Toast (page 55)	Cream Cheese–Stuffed French Toast (leftovers)
Lunch	Chickpea Bolognese (page 91)	Chickpea Bolognese (leftovers)	Lemon Salmon Patties (page 109)	Lemon Salmon Patties (leftovers)	Sweet and Spicy Tofu Stir-Fry (page 92)	Sweet and Spicy Tofu Stir-Fry (leftovers)	Sweet and Spicy-Tofu Stir-Fry (leftovers)
Dinner	Garlic Shrimp Pasta (page 110)	Garlic Shrimp Pasta (leftovers)	Beef Bourguignon (page 129)	Beef Bourguignon (leftovers)	Lemon-Thyme Pork Tenderloin (page 128)	Lemon-Thyme Pork Tenderloin (leftovers)	Cottage Pie (page 124)
Snack	1 clementine and 1 ounce mozzarella cheese	Apple-Cinnamon Oatmeal Muffin (page 59)	Apple-Cinnamon Oatmeal Muffin (leftovers)	4 ounces plain 2% Greek yogurt and 1 clementine	1 small apple and 2 ounces unsalted almonds	Apple-Cinnamon Oatmeal Muffin (leftovers)	4 ounces plain 2% Greek yogurt and 1 clementine

Shopping List

PRODUCE

- Apples (3 small)
- Bell pepper, green (1 medium)
- Blackberries (1 cup)
- Blueberries (1 cup)
- Broccoli florets (1 cup)
- Carrots (2 large)
- Cauliflower head (1 medium)
- Celery stalk (1)
- Clementines (3)
- Garlic head (1)
- Lemon juice (3 ounces)
- Mixed vegetables, frozen (2 cups)
- Mushrooms, white button (1 pint)
- Onion, yellow (1 large)
- Onions, white (2 medium)
- Onions, white (2 small)
- Potato, white (1 small)
- Raspberries (1½ cups)
- Strawberries (1 cup)
- Tomatoes, cherry (12)

DAIRY AND EGGS

- Almond milk, unsweetened plain (1 [64-ounce] carton)
- Cheese, mozzarella (1 ounce)
- Cheese, Parmesan, grated (4 tablespoons)
- Cream cheese, plain (1 [8-ounce] package)
- Eggs (5 large)
- Sour cream (1 [12-ounce] package)
- Yogurt, plain Greek, 2% (1 [32-ounce] container)

MEAT AND SEAFOOD

- Beef sirloin steak (1 pound)
- Beef, ground, 93% lean (8 ounces)
- Pork tenderloin (8 ounces)
- Shrimp, fresh or frozen (1 pound)

PANTRY

- Baking Soda
- Black pepper
- Broth, no-salt-added beef (1 [32-ounce] carton)
- Broth, no-salt-added chicken (1 [32-ounce] carton)

- Chia seeds
- Chickpeas, no-salt-added (1 [15-ounce] can)
- Chili powder
- Cinnamon, ground
- Cooking spray
- Cream of tartar
- Diced tomatoes, no-salt-added (2 [14.5-ounce] cans)
- Flour, all-purpose
- Garlic powder
- Ginger, ground
- Honey
- Oats, old-fashioned rolled
- Olive oil
- Parsley, dried
- Pasta, spaghetti (16 ounces)
- Peaches (1 [15-ounce] can)
- Peanut butter, unsalted
- Pineapple chunks, juice-packed (2 [8-ounce] cans)
- Red pepper flakes
- Rice, parboiled
- Rosemary, dried
- Salmon, skinless and boneless (1 [8-ounce] can)
- Sourdough loaf (1)
- Soy sauce, reduced-sodium
- Thyme, dried
- Tomato paste, no-salt-added (1 [8-ounce] can)
- Vanilla extract
- Vinegar, red wine
- Vinegar, white

OTHER

- Almonds, unsalted
- Applesauce, unsweetened
- Tofu, firm (14 ounces)

Prep Ahead

- Prepare the Stir-Fry Sauce (page 148) for tofu stir-fry ahead of time to let the flavors marinate. This can be kept in the refrigerator for five days.

- Prepare a double batch of High-Protein Oatmeal (page 57), place three servings in the refrigerator for the week, and freeze two servings for later.

- The shopping list will prepare servings for multiple days. Keep two servings available for the meal plan, and freeze extra portions of these recipes for later use: Chickpea Bolognese (page 91), Lemon Salmon Patties (page 109), Garlic Shrimp Pasta (page 110), Beef Bourguignon (page 129), and Lemon-Thyme Pork Tenderloin (page 128). For the Sweet and Spicy Tofu Stir-Fry (page 92), keep three servings available for the meal plan and freeze the extra portion.

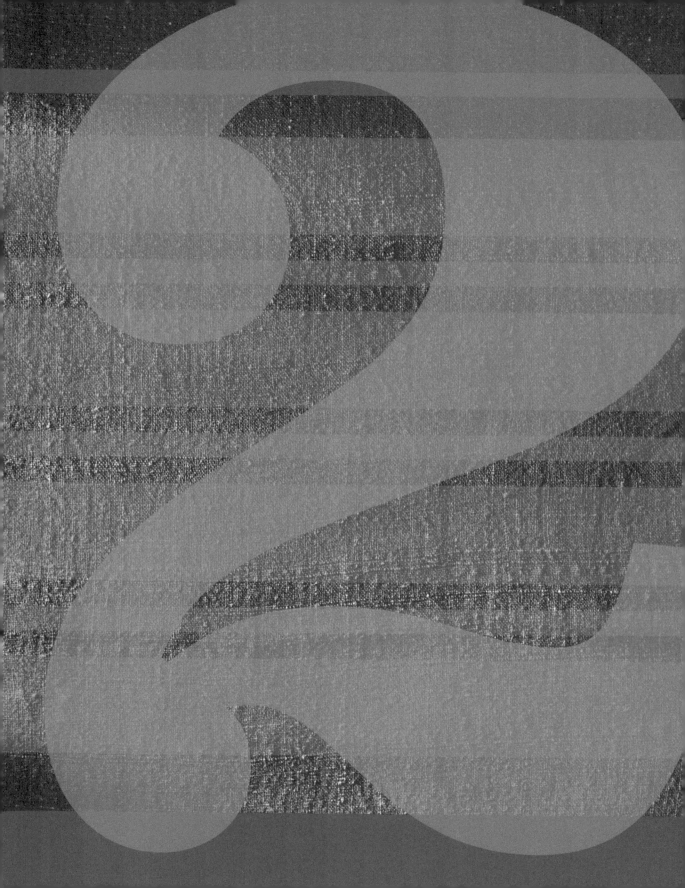

95
Kidney-Friendly
Recipes

THE 95 KIDNEY-FRIENDLY AND EASY-TO-MAKE RECIPES IN this cookbook were developed with you in mind to help support you on your kidney journey with nutritious and delicious foods that can help preserve kidney function. Some recipes include useful tips and information about the foods in the recipe or the preparation method as well as swaps for managing diabetes, cholesterol, or hypertension. At the end of each recipe, a detailed nutrient breakdown per serving is included to help you make informed nutrition choices. Each recipe also contains a label indicating which stage of CKD it's appropriate for, so you can make informed choices about which recipes are right for you. Keep an eye out for the following three labels:

STAGES: ■1–3 ■4 ■5

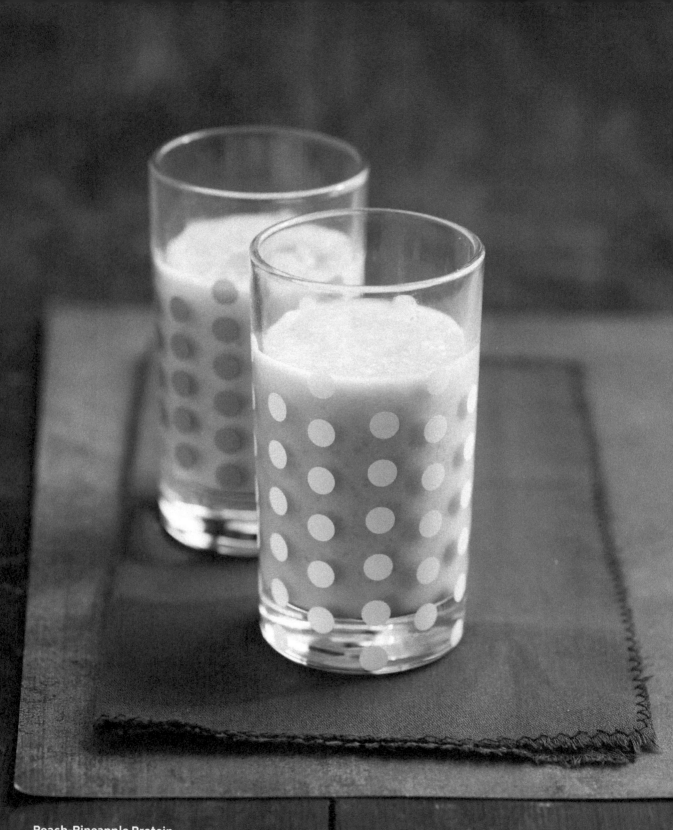

Peach-Pineapple Protein Smoothie, PAGE 56

CHAPTER 3

BREAKFASTS AND SMOOTHIES

Strawberry, Raspberry, and Kale Smoothie ■

PREP TIME: 5 MINUTES • **SERVES** 2

Kefir is a drinkable fermented milk that is a source of probiotics, good bacteria for the digestive tract. Probiotics play an important role in delaying the progression of kidney disease and regulating gut microbiota. The strawberries and raspberries in this smoothie are full of antioxidants and fiber—another benefit.

1 cup plain kefir

½ cup raspberries, fresh or frozen

½ cup chopped raw kale, stemmed

1 cup strawberries, fresh or frozen

1. In a blender, combine the kefir, raspberries, kale, and strawberries and blend until smooth.

2. Pour into glasses and serve immediately.

TIP: Yogurt is a great substitute for the kefir.

Per serving: Calories: 104; Protein: 5g; Total fat: 1.5g; Saturated fat: 0.5g; Total carbohydrates: 19g; Fiber: 3.5g; Cholesterol: 6mg; Phosphorus: 152mg; Potassium: 370mg; Sodium: 49mg; Sugar: 13g

Blueberry, Strawberry, and Cauliflower Smoothie ■

PREP TIME: 5 MINUTES • **SERVES** 2

While it might sound odd, cauliflower is a great low-potassium substitute for bananas in a smoothie. Use fresh or frozen cauliflower to create a smooth and creamy texture. The next time there are extra cauliflower florets on a veggie tray, freeze them to use in this recipe.

½ cup blueberries, fresh or frozen

½ cup sliced strawberries, fresh or frozen

½ cup cauliflower florets

2 tablespoons unsalted peanut butter

1 cup unsweetened plain almond milk

ADAPT FOR DIABETES:

Add extra greens to this smoothie, like ½ cup frozen kale, for extra fiber.

1. In a blender, combine the blueberries, strawberries, cauliflower, peanut butter, and almond milk and blend until smooth.

2. Pour into glasses and serve immediately.

TIP: If potassium is not a concern, also use bananas in this recipe. Try freezing a banana cut into quarters for a quick addition.

Per serving: Calories: 156; Protein: 5g; Total fat: 10g; Saturated fat: 1.5g; Total carbohydrates: 14g; Fiber: 3g; Cholesterol: 0mg; Phosphorus: 93mg; Potassium: 349mg; Sodium: 105mg; Sugar: 8g

Blueberry Pancakes ■

PREP TIME: 5 MINUTES • **COOK TIME:** 10 MINUTES • **SERVES** 4

Pancakes are often one of the foods people with chronic kidney disease are told to avoid. They can be high in phosphorus because of the baking powder used for leavening or the phosphorus additives in convenient boxed mixes. This recipe uses a baking powder substitute (cream of tartar and baking soda) for fluffy, kidney-friendly pancakes.

2 cups all-purpose flour

1 teaspoon cream of tartar

½ teaspoon baking soda

2 teaspoons ground cinnamon

2 cups unsweetened plain almond milk

2 large eggs

1 tablespoon olive oil

Cooking spray

3 cups blueberries, fresh or frozen

1. In a medium bowl, combine the flour, cream of tartar, baking soda, and cinnamon.

2. In a separate bowl, whisk together the almond milk, eggs, and olive oil. Add the dry ingredients and whisk together until combined. Do not overmix.

3. Heat a nonstick skillet over medium heat and spray the skillet with cooking spray.

4. Scoop ⅓ cup of the pancake batter into the skillet. Cook the first side for about 3 minutes, or until bubbles start to form and the underside is brown. Flip, add ⅛ cup of the blueberries to the top of each pancake, and cook on other side for about 2 minutes, or until brown, then remove to a plate and cover to keep warm. Repeat with the remaining batter. You should have a total of 12 pancakes.

Per serving: Calories: 413; Protein: 11g; Total fat: 13g; Saturated fat: 1.5g; Total carbohydrates: 66g; Fiber: 5.5g; Cholesterol: 93mg; Phosphorus: 157mg; Potassium: 486mg; Sodium: 289mg; Sugar: 11g

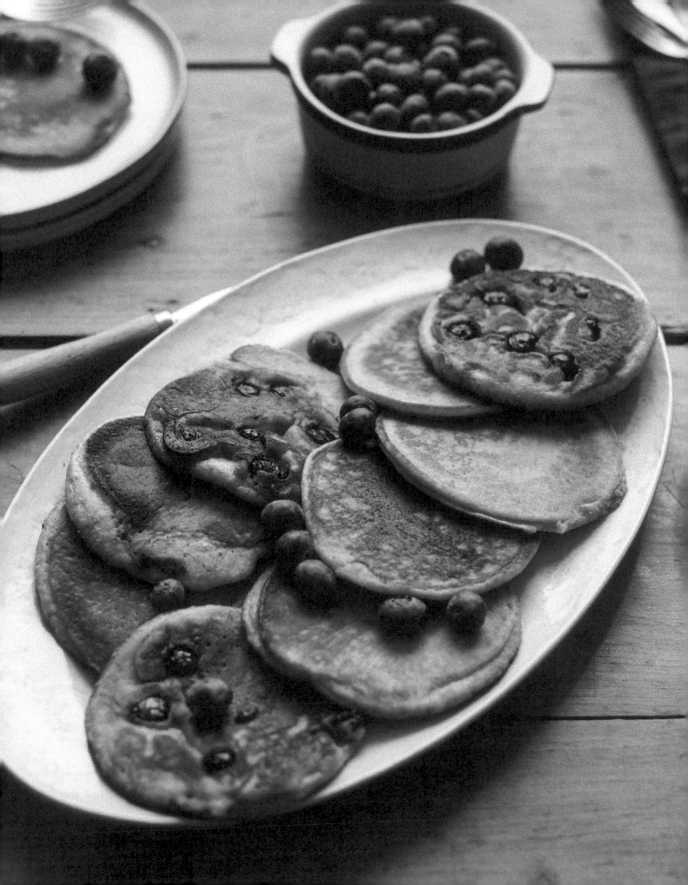

Apple Scone and Yogurt ■

PREP TIME: 10 MINUTES • **COOK TIME:** 20 MINUTES • **SERVES** 4

Apples are a good source of soluble fiber, which can help manage cholesterol and blood glucose levels. They are also a superfood, because they are full of antioxidants and can be enjoyed all year long. These apple scones are quick to prepare and healthier than store-bought options.

2 cups all-purpose flour

¾ teaspoon baking soda

½ teaspoon cream of tartar

4 tablespoons unsalted butter, cold

2 large apples, peeled, cored, and shredded

2 tablespoons honey

½ cup unsweetened plain almond milk

1 teaspoon ground cinnamon

1 cup 2% plain Greek yogurt

ADAPT FOR CARDIOVASCULAR DISEASE:

Use a plant-sterol-enriched margarine for heart-healthy benefits instead of butter.

1. Preheat the oven to 400°F.

2. In a large bowl, mix the flour, baking soda, and cream of tartar.

3. With a pastry cutter or two knives, cut in the butter until the mixture is crumbly.

4. Add the shredded apples, honey, almond milk, and cinnamon to the mixture. Stir to form a soft dough.

5. Place the dough on a clean, dry, lightly floured surface. Knead gently 8 to 10 times with floured hands.

6. Place the dough on a baking sheet and form into a circle roughly 2 inches thick. Use a knife to cut the round of dough into four pie-shaped wedges. Do not cut all the way through the dough to separate the scones.

7. Bake for about 20 minutes, or until lightly browned. Serve immediately with the yogurt.

TIP: Not a fan of apples? Swap out the apples for 1 cup of blueberries, strawberries, or raspberries for an antioxidant boost.

Per serving: Calories: 471; Protein: 13g; Total fat: 14g; Saturated fat: 8g; Total carbohydrates: 75g; Fiber: 4.5g; Cholesterol: 37mg; Phosphorus: 171mg; Potassium: 368mg; Sodium: 285mg; Sugar: 22g

Apple Muesli ■

PREP TIME: 20 MINUTES • **SERVES** 2

Oatmeal is nutritious and delicious, but also extremely versatile. This recipe uses old-fashioned rolled oats, a high-soluble-fiber option that's great for managing cholesterol and blood glucose levels. The old-fashioned rolled oats in this recipe give it a hearty texture and retain more fiber compared to instant oats.

½ cup old-fashioned rolled oats

¾ cup unsweetened plain almond milk

½ cup plain 2% probiotic yogurt

1 teaspoon vanilla extract

2 tablespoons chia seeds

2 teaspoons ground cinnamon

2 small apples, peeled, cored, and chopped

1. In a large bowl, combine the oats, almond milk, yogurt, vanilla, chia seeds, cinnamon, and apples. Stir until well mixed. The mixture will come together like a bowl of oatmeal.

2. Place in the refrigerator for about 15 minutes, or until soft.

3. Serve in a bowl or mason jar. Enjoy cold or warm in the microwave for 30 seconds. Enjoy.

TIP: This recipe can be easily prepared overnight and enjoyed for a quick nutritious and delicious breakfast or snack.

Per serving: Calories: 308; Protein: 12g; Total fat: 8g; Saturated fat: 2g; Total carbohydrates: 50g; Fiber: 11g; Cholesterol: 7mg; Phosphorus: 370mg; Potassium: 644mg; Sodium: 159mg; Sugar: 25g

Cherry Oatmeal ■

PREP TIME: 5 MINUTES • **COOK TIME:** 5 MINUTES • **SERVES** 2

This fiber- and antioxidant-filled breakfast will satisfy until lunch. Cherries provide antioxidants, and the old-fashioned rolled oats are full of fiber. While cherries can be a high-potassium food, the portion size used in this recipe is just enough for flavor and fiber, without too much potassium.

½ cup old-fashioned rolled oats

1 cup unsweetened plain almond milk

½ cup fresh cherries, pitted

2 teaspoons ground cinnamon

1. In a small bowl, combine the oats, almond milk, cherries, and cinnamon.

2. Cook in the microwave for 4 minutes. Remove and stir. The oatmeal will thicken as it cools.

TIP: Add ¼ cup plain probiotic yogurt as a topping to this recipe for a boost of beneficial bacteria for the gut and an extra-creamy taste.

Per serving: Calories: 125; Protein: 4g; Total fat: 3g; Saturated fat: 0g; Total carbohydrates: 23g; Fiber: 4g; Cholesterol: 0mg; Phosphorus: 98mg; Potassium: 259mg; Sodium: 93mg; Sugar: 5.5g

Baked Eggs Shakshuka ■

PREP TIME: 15 MINUTES • **COOK TIME:** 30 MINUTES • **SERVES** 4

There is something very comforting about mixed eggs, tomatoes, and spices. Known as shakshuka, a classic North African and Middle Eastern dish, this recipe will certainly wake up the taste buds. This baked egg dish is great for a weekend brunch or a holiday celebration.

½ teaspoon ground cumin

½ teaspoon paprika

1 teaspoon dried thyme

1 tablespoon olive oil

1 small white onion, sliced

1 garlic clove, minced

2 medium red bell peppers, sliced

3 ripe medium Roma tomatoes, chopped

4 large eggs

4 small slices sourdough bread

ADAPT FOR DIABETES:

Choose low-glycemic-index and kidney-friendly breads like sourdough, 60% whole wheat, or light rye.

1. Preheat the oven to 400°F.

2. In a medium ovenproof sauté pan or cast-iron skillet over medium-high heat, toast the cumin, paprika, and thyme for about 1 minute, until fragrant. Add the olive oil, onion, garlic, and bell peppers and cook for about 5 minutes, stirring often, until the vegetables are soft.

3. Add the tomatoes, reduce the heat to medium, and let simmer for 10 minutes, stirring once or twice.

4. Make four craters in the tomato mixture and carefully crack an egg into each crater. Transfer the pan to the oven and bake for about 15 minutes, or until the egg whites are opaque and the yolks have risen a bit but are still soft. Or cook to preference.

5. Serve immediately with a slice of the sourdough bread and enjoy.

TIP: This recipe would easily double as a delicious dinner option on a cold day with a side salad.

Per serving: Calories: 226; Protein: 11g; Total fat: 9.5g; Saturated fat: 2g; Total carbohydrates: 25g; Fiber: 3g; Cholesterol: 186mg; Phosphorus: 167mg; Potassium: 379mg; Sodium: 270mg; Sugar: 6g

Blueberry-Lentil Muffins ■

PREP TIME: 10 MINUTES • **COOK TIME:** 20 MINUTES • **MAKES** 12 MUFFINS

Don't let the lentils in this blueberry muffin concern you. They aren't even noticeable by taste, but they add a stealthy boost of protein and fiber and are a great plant-based protein. This recipe uses canned lentils for convenience, but they are also a lower-potassium option compared to dried beans. These muffins are great as a grab-and-go item.

Cooking spray

1 cup canned lentils, no added salt, drained

½ cup water

1 large egg

½ cup olive oil

½ cup unsweetened applesauce

1 teaspoon vanilla extract

1⅓ cups all-purpose flour

⅓ teaspoon baking soda

¾ teaspoon cream of tartar

2 cups blueberries

ADAPT FOR HYPERTENSION:

Add an extra ½ cup raspberries for a burst of antioxidants.

1. Preheat the oven to 400°F. Spray a 12-cup muffin tin with cooking spray.

2. In a food processor or blender, puree the lentils and water until smooth. Scrape the puree into a large bowl.

3. Combine the egg, olive oil, applesauce, and vanilla with the lentil puree.

4. Add the flour, baking soda, and cream of tartar to the egg mixture and combine.

5. Mix in the blueberries.

6. Portion into the prepared muffin tin, filling each cup about two-thirds full.

7. Bake in the oven for 15 to 20 minutes, until a toothpick inserted in the center comes out clean. Remove from the oven and let cool before eating.

TIP: To increase the potassium content, add 1 mashed banana to this recipe.

TIP: Store the muffins on the counter in an airtight container for 3 days. Warm them in the microwave for 15 seconds before enjoying.

Per serving (1 muffin): Calories: 184; Protein: 4g; Total fat: 11g; Saturated fat: 1.5g; Total carbohydrates: 19g; Fiber: 2.5g; Cholesterol: 15mg; Phosphorus: 55mg; Potassium: 137mg; Sodium: 73mg; Sugar: 4g

Lemon and Red Pepper Avocado Toast ■

PREP TIME: 5 MINUTES • **COOK TIME:** 5 MINUTES • **SERVES** 4

People with chronic kidney disease often avoid avocado because of its high potassium content. Even on a potassium restriction, this perfectly portioned avocado toast will be sure to please. This recipe is a great example of how favorite foods eaten in moderation can still be healthy.

4 large eggs

1 teaspoon freshly ground black pepper

1 small avocado

2 tablespoons lemon juice

2 teaspoons red pepper flakes

4 small slices sourdough bread, toasted

16 grape tomatoes sliced in half

1. In a medium nonstick pan over medium heat, cook the eggs sunny-side up for about 3 minutes, or until the whites are mostly set, with some still-runny whites near the yolks. Season with the pepper.

2. In a small bowl, mash together the avocado, lemon juice, and red pepper flakes.

3. Top the toasted bread with the avocado mixture and 4 tomato halves per slice. Top with the egg and serve immediately.

TIP: Make this a high-protein option for stage 5 by adding an additional egg per serving.

Per serving: Calories: 225; Protein: 11g; Total fat: 10g; Saturated fat: 2.5g; Total carbohydrates: 24g; Fiber: 4g; Cholesterol: 186mg; Phosphorus: 169mg; Potassium: 448mg; Sodium: 270mg; Sugar: 4g

Berry and Chia Seed Pudding ■

PREP TIME: 20 MINUTES • **SERVES** 2

Chia seeds contain fiber and omega-3 fatty acids, both of which are great for chronic kidney disease, heart disease, and diabetes. When chia seeds are mixed with almond milk, they make a sort of pudding that takes on the flavor of fruit eaten with it.

¼ cup chia seeds

1 cup unsweetened plain almond milk

1 teaspoon vanilla extract

½ teaspoon ground cinnamon

1 cup halved strawberries

1 cup raspberries

ADAPT FOR DIABETES:

Top the pudding with extra chia seeds or flax-seed for an extra source of fiber and crunch.

1. In a small bowl, mix the chia seeds, almond milk, vanilla, and cinnamon.

2. Let the mixture sit for about 15 minutes in the refrigerator. It is ready when it has a pudding-like texture.

3. Serve immediately topped with the strawberries and raspberries.

TIP: Substitute ground chia seeds for whole seeds in this recipe for a smoother texture. Double the amount of chia seeds if using ground.

Per serving: Calories: 188; Protein: 6g; Total fat: 8.5g; Saturated fat: 1g; Total carbohydrates: 24g; Fiber: 13g; Cholesterol: 0mg; Phosphorus: 232mg; Potassium: 399mg; Sodium: 98mg; Sugar: 7g

Cream Cheese–Stuffed French Toast ■

PREP TIME: 10 MINUTES • **COOK TIME:** 15 MINUTES • **SERVES** 2

This recipe is a bit of comfort food with a touch of class. It's for celebrations or a way to impress guests. Cream cheese is a low-phosphorus, kidney-friendly cheese option. Try using different flavors of cream cheese, like strawberry, to spice up this recipe.

2 large eggs

1 teaspoon vanilla extract

1 teaspoon ground cinnamon

4 small slices sourdough bread

¼ cup plain cream cheese

½ cup raspberries, mashed

Cooking spray

1 cup strawberries, halved

1. In a medium bowl, whisk together the eggs, vanilla, and cinnamon. Set aside.

2. Spread two slices of bread with the cream cheese and then top each slice with the raspberries. Top with the remaining two slices of bread to form two sandwiches.

3. Dip the sandwiches in the egg mixture to coat completely.

4. Heat a nonstick skillet over medium-high heat and spray the skillet with cooking spray. Cook the sandwiches until golden brown on both sides, or use a sandwich press to cook.

5. Top with the strawberries and serve immediately.

Per serving: Calories: 395; Protein: 16g; Total fat: 17g; Saturated fat: 8g; Total carbohydrates: 46g; Fiber: 5.5g; Cholesterol: 215mg; Phosphorus: 224mg; Potassium: 347mg; Sodium: 549mg; Sugar: 9.5g

Peach-Pineapple Protein Smoothie ■

PREP TIME: 5 MINUTES • **SERVES** 2

This protein-packed smoothie can be prepared the night before and stored in the refrigerator for a quick and speedy breakfast. Using canned fruit in this recipe is a healthy and safe way to get peaches onto the taste buds. Peaches usually have higher amounts of potassium, but the potassium leaches out of the fruit during the canning process.

1 (15-ounce) can peaches, drained

2 (8-ounce) cans juice-packed pineapple chunks, drained

½ cup 2% plain Greek yogurt

1 cup unsweetened plain almond milk

1 tablespoon chia seeds

1. Add the peaches, pineapple, yogurt, almond milk, and chia seeds to a blender and blend until smooth.

2. Pour into glasses and serve immediately.

TIP: For variety, you can substitute strawberries or blueberries. Fresh or frozen fruit can be used instead of canned.

Per serving: Calories: 235; Protein: 10g; Total fat: 4.5g; Saturated fat: 1g; Total carbohydrates: 44g; Fiber: 5g; Cholesterol: 6mg; Phosphorus: 184mg; Potassium: 574mg; Sodium: 124mg; Sugar: 36g

High-Protein Oatmeal ■

PREP TIME: 5 MINUTES • **COOK TIME:** 10 MINUTES • **SERVES** 2

A balanced breakfast does not need to be complicated. This protein-packed breakfast has all the food groups and gives a burst of energy, protein, and fiber. Oats are incredibly nutritious as a source of antioxidants and soluble fiber.

1 cup unsweetened plain almond milk

½ cup 2% plain Greek yogurt

2 tablespoons unsalted peanut butter

1 teaspoon vanilla extract

1 cup old-fashioned rolled oats

½ cup blueberries

½ cup blackberries

½ cup raspberries

ADAPT FOR CARDIOVASCULAR DISEASE:

Use low-fat Greek yogurt.

1. In a small bowl, mix the almond milk, yogurt, peanut butter, vanilla, and oats until well blended.

2. Split into two bowls or mason jars and divide the berries between each bowl or jar.

3. Microwave for 4 minutes. Remove from the microwave and stir. The oatmeal will thicken as it cools.

TIP: Lower the protein in this recipe by swapping out the Greek yogurt for regular yogurt. Individuals in stages 1 to 4 should be following a low-protein diet.

Per serving: Calories: 369; Protein: 17g; Total fat: 14g; Saturated fat: 3g; Total carbohydrates: 46g; Fiber: 9.5g; Cholesterol: 6mg; Phosphorus: 322mg; Potassium: 550mg; Sodium: 118mg; Sugar: 12g

Arugula, Pepper, and Onion Egg Cups ■

PREP TIME: 5 MINUTES • **COOK TIME:** 25 MINUTES • **SERVES** 4

These eggs are perfect for preparing ahead of time and using throughout the week as a great grab-and-go breakfast item. Adding extra vegetables like bell peppers and arugula provides a pop of color and extra fiber.

Cooking spray

8 large eggs

2 tablespoons unsweetened plain almond milk

½ teaspoon onion powder

½ teaspoon garlic powder

¼ teaspoon freshly ground black pepper

½ teaspoon dried parsley

½ cup chopped red bell pepper

½ cup chopped yellow bell pepper

1 cup arugula

ADAPT FOR HIGH CHOLESTEROL:

Swap out 4 of the eggs for ½ cup egg whites for a lower-cholesterol option.

1. Preheat the oven to 350°F and spray 8 cups of a muffin tin with cooking spray.

2. In a medium bowl, beat the eggs, almond milk, onion powder, garlic powder, pepper, and parsley together.

3. Divide the red and yellow peppers and arugula among the prepared muffin cups. Pour the egg mixture over, leaving space at the top for the egg to rise.

4. Bake in the oven for 18 to 22 minutes, until the eggs become opaque and the yolks have risen a bit but are still soft.

TIP: Store the egg cups in an airtight container in the refrigerator for 1 day (reheat in the microwave for 25 to 30 seconds), or in the freezer for 3 days (reheat in the microwave for 50 to 60 seconds).

Per serving: Calories: 189; Protein: 13g; Total fat: 14g; Saturated fat: 3g; Total carbohydrates: 4g; Fiber: 0.5g; Cholesterol: 372mg; Phosphorus: 210mg; Potassium: 219mg; Sodium: 153mg; Sugar: 1.5g

Apple-Cinnamon Oatmeal Muffins ◾

PREP TIME: 10 MINUTES • **COOK TIME:** 20 MINUTES • **MAKES** 12 MUFFINS

Muffin comes from the French word "moufflet," a term that is often applied to bread and means soft. Old-fashioned rolled oats and chia seeds add extra fiber to maintain fullness for longer.

Cooking spray

2 large eggs

2 tablespoons honey

½ cup unsweetened applesauce

½ cup olive oil

2 teaspoons vanilla extract

1½ cups all-purpose flour

1 teaspoon Baking Powder Substitute (page 146)

2 teaspoons ground cinnamon

2 tablespoons chia seeds

½ cup old-fashioned rolled oats

1½ cups peeled, cored, and chopped apples

ADAPT FOR DIABETES:

Replace the honey with an extra 2 tablespoons of unsweetened applesauce for a lower-carbohydrate option.

1. Preheat the oven to 400°F and spray a 12-cup muffin tin with cooking spray.

2. In a large bowl, whisk together the eggs, honey, applesauce, olive oil, and vanilla.

3. In another large bowl, combine the flour, Baking Powder Substitute, cinnamon, chia seeds, and oats.

4. Fold the wet ingredients into the dry ingredients. Add the apples and mix.

5. Fill each muffin cup three-quarters full. Bake in the oven for about 20 minutes, or until a toothpick inserted in the center comes out clean. Cool and remove from muffin tins. Serve warm.

TIP: Chia seeds are a great omega-3 addition to the muffins. If potassium is not a concern, hemp hearts can be sprinkled on top before baking.

TIP: Store the muffins on the counter in an airtight container for 3 days. If freezing to enjoy later, let the muffins thaw completely on the counter, or reheat in the microwave for 30 to 60 seconds.

Per serving (1 muffin): Calories: 206; Protein: 3g; Total fat: 12g; Saturated fat: 1.5g; Total carbohydrates: 22g; Fiber: 2g; Cholesterol: 31mg; Phosphorus: 64mg; Potassium: 77mg; Sodium: 118mg; Sugar: 5.5g

Tangy Garlic-Roasted
Brussels Sprouts, PAGE 63

SIDES AND SNACKS

Sweet and Savory
Mashed Squash and Carrots ■

PREP TIME: 5 MINUTES • **COOK TIME:** 20 MINUTES • **SERVES** 8

Don't be worried about the addition of squash if potassium is a concern. This recipe uses spaghetti squash, a lower-potassium option compared to other squash varieties. When pureed with carrots, it provides a smooth and savory fall-inspired dish.

1 small spaghetti squash

2½ cups peeled, chopped carrots

1 tablespoon honey

½ teaspoon ground cinnamon

½ teaspoon paprika

2 tablespoons unsalted butter

ADAPT FOR DIABETES:

This recipe is sweet enough. Leave out the honey.

1. Place the squash in the microwave and cook on high for 5 minutes. This makes the squash easier to cut through.

2. Cut the squash in half lengthwise and scrape out the seeds with a spoon. Place the squash halves, cut-side down, in a medium microwave-safe dish with about a half inch of water in the bottom of the dish. Microwave on high for 10 to 15 minutes, until the squash is fork-tender.

3. Fill a medium pot with water and bring to a boil on high heat. Once at a boil, add the carrots and lower the heat to a simmer. Cook the carrots until fork-tender, about 10 minutes.

4. Once the carrots and squash are cooked, transfer the vegetables to a blender or food processor and mix until smooth. Mix in the honey, cinnamon, paprika, and butter.

TIP: Looking for a high-potassium option? Swap out the spaghetti squash for butternut or acorn squash.

Per serving: Calories: 88; Protein: 1g; Total fat: 3.5g; Saturated fat: 2g; Total carbohydrates: 14g; Fiber: 3g; Cholesterol: 8mg; Phosphorus: 30mg; Potassium: 265mg; Sodium: 49mg; Sugar: 7g

Tangy Garlic-Roasted Brussels Sprouts ■

PREP TIME: 5 MINUTES • **COOK TIME:** 25 MINUTES • **SERVES** 4

Brussels sprouts are a cruciferous vegetable related to broccoli and cabbage and are a antioxidant and fiber-rich vegetable. These aren't typical Brussels sprouts. The red wine vinegar adds a tangy and sweet spin to this classic dish.

1 tablespoon olive oil

2 tablespoons red wine vinegar, divided

½ tablespoon garlic powder

¼ teaspoon freshly ground black pepper

2 cups Brussels sprouts, halved

ADAPT FOR HYPERTENSION:

Add 2 tablespoons of chopped macadamia nuts for a source of heart-healthy fats.

1. Preheat the oven to 450°F. Cover a baking sheet with aluminum foil and set aside.

2. Whisk together the olive oil, 1 tablespoon of vinegar, the garlic powder, and pepper. Coat the Brussels sprouts with the olive oil and vinegar mixture and spread the sprouts out evenly over the prepared baking sheet.

3. Roast in the oven for 20 to 25 minutes, until the sprouts are tender-crisp.

4. Drizzle with the remaining 1 tablespoon of vinegar before serving.

Per serving: Calories: 54; Protein: 2g; Total fat: 3.5g; Saturated fat: 0.5g; Total carbohydrates: 5g; Fiber: 2g; Cholesterol: 0mg; Phosphorus: 36mg; Potassium: 190mg; Sodium: 12mg; Sugar: 1g

Homestyle Coleslaw with Apples ■

PREP TIME: 10 MINUTES • **SERVES** 8

Raw cabbage is the only consistent item in this new take on a coleslaw mix, while the apples provide a sweetness to this traditional tasty dish. Cabbage belongs to the same family as broccoli and cauliflower and is full of vitamins, antioxidants, and fiber. Cabbage may help with inflammation and improve digestion.

3 cups shredded green cabbage

1 cup shredded red cabbage

1 medium green apple, peeled, cored, and chopped

1 medium red apple, peeled, cored, and chopped

1 cup shredded carrots

2 scallions, chopped (white and green parts)

⅓ cup 2% plain Greek yogurt

1 tablespoon honey

1 tablespoon lemon juice

1 tablespoon white vinegar

ADAPT FOR HIGH CHOLESTEROL:

Replace the Greek yogurt with plain, low-fat yogurt.

1. In a large bowl, combine the green and red cabbage, green and red apples, carrots, and scallions.

2. In a small bowl, mix the yogurt, honey, lemon juice, and vinegar. Pour the dressing over the cabbage slaw. Enjoy right away or let sit in the refrigerator for 15 minutes for the flavors to soak in.

TIP: Leftovers can be stored in the refrigerator in an airtight container for up to 2 days.

Per serving: Calories: 42; Protein: 2g; Total fat: 0g; Saturated fat: 0g; Total carbohydrates: 9g; Fiber: 2g; Cholesterol: 1mg; Phosphorus: 21mg; Potassium: 74mg; Sodium: 17mg; Sugar: 6.5g

Crunchy Cauliflower Salad ■

PREP TIME: 35 MINUTES • **COOK TIME:** 10 MINUTES • **SERVES** 8

Cauliflower, meaning cabbage flower, is a delicate vegetable to grow, but it provides a lot of antioxidants and fiber to a diet. This tangy salad absorbs the flavors of the garlic, red pepper flakes, and vinegar and makes a crunchy side dish.

1 medium cauliflower head, chopped into florets

1 tablespoon garlic powder

1 teaspoon freshly ground black pepper

1 teaspoon red pepper flakes

3 tablespoons white vinegar

6 tablespoons olive oil

1. Add one inch of water to a large pot and place a steamer basket inside. Bring the water to a boil, add the cauliflower to the steamer basket, cover, and steam for 6 minutes. The cauliflower should be fork-tender but still maintain its shape. Drain and rinse with cold water.

2. In a large bowl, mix the garlic powder, pepper, red pepper flakes, vinegar, and olive oil. Add the cauliflower and toss together.

3. Marinate the cauliflower for 30 minutes in the refrigerator before serving cold.

TIP: If a steamer basket isn't available, place the cauliflower directly in 1 to 2 inches of water to cook.

Per serving: Calories: 114; Protein: 2g; Total fat: 10g; Saturated fat: 1.5g; Total carbohydrates: 5g; Fiber: 1.5g; Cholesterol: 0mg; Phosphorus: 38mg; Potassium: 242mg; Sodium: 23mg; Sugar: 1.5g

Garlic Double-Boiled Mashed Potatoes ■

PREP TIME: 5 MINUTES • **COOK TIME:** 15 MINUTES • **SERVES** 4

Potatoes are considered a staple food in the United States but are often not recommended for those who have CKD due to their high potassium content. Double boiling potatoes and other root vegetables reduces the potassium by 50 percent. They will still have a lot of potassium, so keep portions to ½-cup servings. These smooth and creamy garlic mashed potatoes are warm and inviting.

2 medium white potatoes (480g total), peeled and cut into 1-inch pieces

1 tablespoon unsalted butter

1 teaspoon garlic powder

½ teaspoon onion powder

½ teaspoon dried parsley

ADAPT FOR DIABETES:

Choose sweet potatoes for a low-glycemic-index choice.

1. Place the potatoes in a large pot with 4 inches of water above the potatoes. Boil for 5 minutes; the potatoes will not be tender. Drain the water and refill with fresh water 4 inches above the potatoes. Boil again until the potatoes are tender, about 10 minutes.

2. Drain and discard the water. Return the potatoes to the pot.

3. Add the butter to the pot and mash the potatoes.

4. Mix in the garlic powder, onion powder, and parsley and enjoy.

TIP: Double-boiled potatoes can be roasted or mashed after cooking.

Per serving: Calories: 112; Protein: 2g; Total fat: 3g; Saturated fat: 2g; Total carbohydrates: 20g; Fiber: 3g; Cholesterol: 8mg; Phosphorus: 80mg; Potassium: 259mg; Sodium: 21mg; Sugar: 1.5g

Honey-Vanilla Energy Balls ■

PREP TIME: 10 MINUTES, PLUS 1 HOUR TO CHILL • **MAKES** 20 ENERGY BALLS

In the afternoon when that drop in energy hits and the craving for something sweet starts, these delicious energy treats will help. These little balls are perfect for packing up and carrying for a snack later. With the addition of peanut butter and chia seeds for protein, that full feeling will stick around longer.

1½ cups old-fashioned rolled oats

½ cup unsalted peanut butter

¼ cup honey

1½ teaspoons vanilla extract

2 tablespoons chia seeds

1. Line a pan or baking sheet with parchment paper.

2. In a large bowl, combine the oats, peanut butter, honey, vanilla, and chia seeds.

3. Roll into 20 balls approximately 1 inch in diameter each, and place on the prepared baking sheet.

4. Chill for 1 hour in the refrigerator.

TIP: Dried unsweetened cranberries make a great addition to this recipe.

TIP: Leftovers can be stored in an airtight container for up to 3 days in the refrigerator.

Per serving (2 energy balls): Calories: 318; Protein: 9g; Total fat: 16g; Saturated fat: 3g; Total carbohydrates: 37g; Fiber: 5g; Cholesterol: 0mg; Phosphorus: 213mg; Potassium: 260mg; Sodium: 6mg; Sugar: 16g

Spicy Buffalo Cauliflower Bites ■

PREP TIME: 5 MINUTES • **COOK TIME:** 40 MINUTES • **SERVES** 12

This is a great kidney-friendly snack or appetizer. These baked cauliflower bites are high in fiber and low in sodium, but just as spicy and delicious as wings. The cauliflower pieces turn crispy, and the homemade Buffalo sauce provides an awesome coating that makes these a spicy and tangy snack.

½ cup water

½ cup all-purpose flour

2 tablespoons garlic powder

1 teaspoon freshly ground black pepper

1 small cauliflower head, cut into bite-size pieces

¼ cup Buffalo Hot Sauce (page 155)

¾ cup Rosemary-Garlic Sauce (page 154)

1. Preheat the oven to 450°F. Line a baking sheet with parchment paper.

2. In a medium bowl, combine the water, flour, garlic powder, and pepper and stir well until combined.

3. Coat the cauliflower pieces in the flour mixture. Place on the prepared baking sheet and roast in the oven, tossing halfway through the cooking, for about 20 minutes, or until the bites are golden brown and crunchy.

4. Remove the cauliflower from the oven, place in a large bowl, and toss to coat with the hot sauce. Place the cauliflower back on the baking sheet and continue baking for 15 to 20 minutes, until crispy.

5. Remove the cauliflower from the oven and let sit for 10 minutes before serving. Serve warm with the Rosemary-Garlic Sauce.

TIP: No time to make the Buffalo Hot Sauce? No worries, a premade option, like Frank's RedHot, can be used. Be sure to compare food labels for the lowest-sodium option.

Per serving: Calories: 34; Protein: 1g; Total fat: 0.5g; Saturated fat: 0g; Total carbohydrates: 7g; Fiber: 1g; Cholesterol: 0mg; Phosphorus: 24mg; Potassium: 102mg; Sodium: 20mg; Sugar: 0.5g

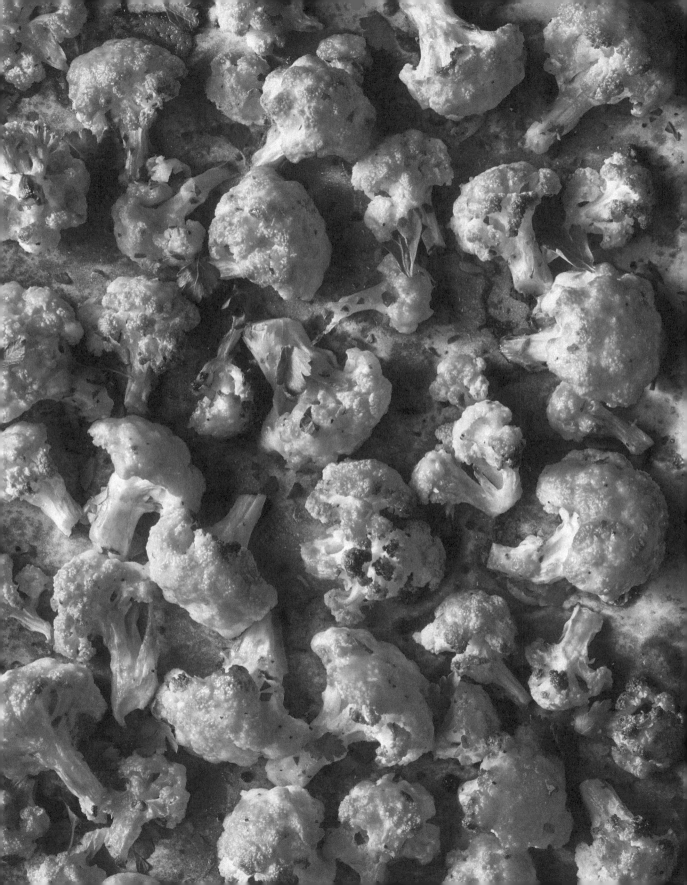

Roasted Carrots and Leeks ■

PREP TIME: 5 MINUTES • **COOK TIME:** 30 MINUTES • **SERVES** 4

This super-easy dish is a tender and flavorful companion for any protein. Carrots and leeks are great sources of fiber and vitamin C and are available year-round.

2 tablespoons olive oil

1 tablespoon white vinegar

1 tablespoon honey

1 teaspoon dried thyme

1 teaspoon freshly ground black pepper

6 medium carrots, peeled and sliced into coins

3 leeks, chopped, white and light green parts

1. Preheat the oven to 375°F. Line a baking sheet with aluminum foil and set aside.

2. In a small bowl, whisk together the olive oil, vinegar, honey, thyme, and pepper. Coat the carrots and leeks with the oil-and-vinegar mixture, and spread the vegetables evenly on the prepared baking sheet.

3. Roast in the oven, tossing halfway through cooking, for 30 minutes, or until the carrots are tender-crisp.

TIP: Parsnips are a great high-potassium addition to this recipe.

Per serving: Calories: 157; Protein: 2g; Total fat: 7g; Saturated fat: 1g; Total carbohydrates: 23g; Fiber: 4g; Cholesterol: 0mg; Phosphorus: 57mg; Potassium: 425mg; Sodium: 77mg; Sugar: 11g

Baba Ghanoush Dip ■

PREP TIME: 10 MINUTES • **COOK TIME:** 30 MINUTES • **SERVES** 8

Baba ghanoush is a Middle Eastern dip made with charred eggplant (also called an aubergine). Eggplant is a high-fiber fruit similar to tomatoes and peppers. In this recipe, the eggplant is roasted as a quick time-saver instead of charring. The ingredients of this dish come together for a smooth, creamy, tangy, and spicy dip that can be enjoyed as an appetizer with pita bread or veggies or as a condiment on sandwiches.

2 medium
  eggplants, halved

2 garlic cloves

¼ teaspoon
  ground cumin

¼ teaspoon paprika

1 tablespoon lemon juice

1. Preheat the oven to 400°F. Roast the eggplants for about 30 minutes, or until the interior is very tender and the skin is collapsing and a deep dark purple.

2. Scoop out the flesh of the eggplants with a large spoon, leaving the skin behind.

3. In a high-speed blender or food processor, combine the eggplant flesh, garlic, cumin, paprika, and lemon juice and mix until smooth.

4. Serve immediately or store in the refrigerator in an airtight container for 2 days.

Per serving: Calories: 36; Protein: 1g; Total fat: 0g; Saturated fat: 0g; Total carbohydrates: 8g; Fiber: 4g; Cholesterol: 0mg; Phosphorus: 34mg; Potassium: 320mg; Sodium: 3mg; Sugar: 4.5g

Fruit Dip ■

With hints of vanilla and cinnamon, this crowd-pleaser is great for entertaining. A great replacement for store-bought dip, this is easy to make and can be stored in the refrigerator for snacks or lunches. Use your favorite fruits, choosing low-potassium options such as blueberries, pineapple, strawberries, and apple slices.

1 cup plain cream cheese, softened

1 cup plain low-fat probiotic yogurt

1 teaspoon vanilla extract

1 tablespoon lemon juice

1 tablespoon ground cinnamon

Cut fruit of your choice, for serving

1. In a blender or food processor, mix the cream cheese, yogurt, vanilla, lemon juice, and cinnamon until well combined.

2. Place the cream cheese mixture in small bowl and chill, covered, in the refrigerator for 45 minutes.

3. Remove and serve with the fruit of your choice.

TIP: Store leftovers in the refrigerator in an airtight container for 2 days.

Per serving: Calories: 97; Protein: 2g; Total fat: 7g; Saturated fat: 4g; Total carbohydrates: 7g; Fiber: 1g; Cholesterol: 21mg; Phosphorus: 54mg; Potassium: 97mg; Sodium: 75mg; Sugar: 4.5g

Chili Roasted Broccoli ■

PREP TIME: 5 MINUTES • **COOK TIME:** 15 MINUTES • **SERVES** 4

Roasting broccoli takes this cruciferous veggie to an entirely new level. Roasting allows the broccoli to stay crisp and crunchy while taking on the flavors it's seasoned with. Using herbs in this recipe is a low-sodium way of flavoring foods.

3 cups broccoli florets

1 tablespoon olive oil

½ teaspoon chili powder

¼ teaspoon ground cumin

1 tablespoon lemon juice

1. Preheat the oven to 425°F. Line a baking sheet with aluminum foil.

2. In a medium bowl, toss the broccoli florets with the olive oil, chili powder, and cumin until coated.

3. Place the broccoli on the prepared baking sheet and roast for 8 to 12 minutes, until fork-tender and lightly brown.

4. Toss with the lemon juice and serve.

TIP: Any dried herb can be used to season roasted broccoli. Try onion powder and freshly ground black pepper for another low-sodium option.

Per serving: Calories: 46; Protein: 2g; Total fat: 3.5g; Saturated fat: 0.5g; Total carbohydrates: 3g; Fiber: 1g; Cholesterol: 0mg; Phosphorus: 35mg; Potassium: 177mg; Sodium: 17mg; Sugar: 1g

Lemon-Garlic Green Beans ■

PREP TIME: 5 MINUTES • **COOK TIME:** 5 MINUTES • **SERVES** 6

Green beans are often also called string beans or snap beans and come in a variety of colors like green, yellow, purple, or even speckled. This recipe uses green beans, but other colors can be used instead. Blanching green beans softens and cooks them while also retaining most of the vitamins because of the short cooking time.

3 cups green beans

1 tablespoon olive oil

2 tablespoons garlic powder

1 teaspoon red pepper flakes

1 tablespoon lemon juice

½ teaspoon freshly ground black pepper

1. In a pot of boiling water, blanch the green beans for 2 minutes. Drain and place in cold water for 1 minute to stop the cooking. Remove from the cold water and pat dry.

2. In a small bowl, whisk together the olive oil, garlic powder, red pepper flakes, lemon juice, and pepper.

3. In a large bowl, combine the olive oil mixture and green beans until the beans are well coated.

4. Enjoy at room temperature.

TIP: Blanching is a cooking method where food is scalded in boiling water, removed after a short period of time, then placed in ice water to stop the cooking process. Blanching foods helps retain vitamins and keeps vegetables crisp. Try blanching peas, broccoli, cauliflower, or cabbage.

Per serving: Calories: 48; Protein: 1g; Total fat: 2.5g; Saturated fat: 0.5g; Total carbohydrates: 6g; Fiber: 2g; Cholesterol: 0mg; Phosphorus: 33mg; Potassium: 154mg; Sodium: 5mg; Sugar: 2g

Mediterranean Marinated Chickpea Salad ■

PREP TIME: 15 MINUTES • **SERVES** 8

Beans and legumes are a great addition to a kidney-friendly diet, and using canned beans helps reduce the potassium content—just look for no-added-salt products. Chickpeas or garbanzo beans are a great source of iron and fiber.

2 teaspoons
ground cumin

1 teaspoon paprika

2 teaspoons
garlic powder

2 tablespoons
lemon juice

1 tablespoon olive oil

½ teaspoon white vinegar

2 (15-ounce) cans
chickpeas, no added
salt, drained and rinsed

½ cup chopped green
bell pepper

¼ cup chopped red onion

1. In a large bowl, mix the cumin, paprika, garlic powder, lemon juice, olive oil, and vinegar to make the dressing.

2. Add the chickpeas, bell pepper, and red onion to the dressing and toss together until well coated.

TIP: This salad keeps well in the refrigerator in an airtight container for up to 3 days.

Per serving: Calories: 117; Protein: 6g; Total fat: 4g; Saturated fat: 0.5g; Total carbohydrates: 16g; Fiber: 5g; Cholesterol: 0mg; Phosphorus: 92mg; Potassium: 195mg; Sodium: 141mg; Sugar: 3.5g

Garlic Hummus ▪

PREP TIME: 10 MINUTES • **MAKES** 2½ CUPS

This legume dip takes on the refreshing flavors of the spices and lemon, and provides fiber and protein. Enjoy with crackers or vegetables. Traditionally hummus is made with a base of chickpeas and tahini, but this lower-phosphorus option is just as creamy without the tahini. For extra texture, keep some chickpeas aside to top the hummus with before serving.

2 (15-ounce) cans chickpeas, no added salt, drained

¼ cup lemon juice

4 garlic cloves, finely chopped

1 tablespoon paprika

½ teaspoon ground cumin

¼ teaspoon salt

2 teaspoons extra virgin olive oil

1. In a blender combine the chickpeas, lemon juice, garlic, paprika, cumin, and salt. Process until smooth.

2. Drizzle with olive oil and serve immediately, or store in the refrigerator in an airtight container for 3 days.

TIP: Hummus can make a great addition to veggie sandwiches or wraps.

Per serving (¼ cup): Calories: 77; Protein: 4g; Total fat: 2.5g; Saturated fat: 0g; Total carbohydrates: 11g; Fiber: 3.5g; Cholesterol: 0mg; Phosphorus: 62mg; Potassium: 131mg; Sodium: 154mg; Sugar: 2g

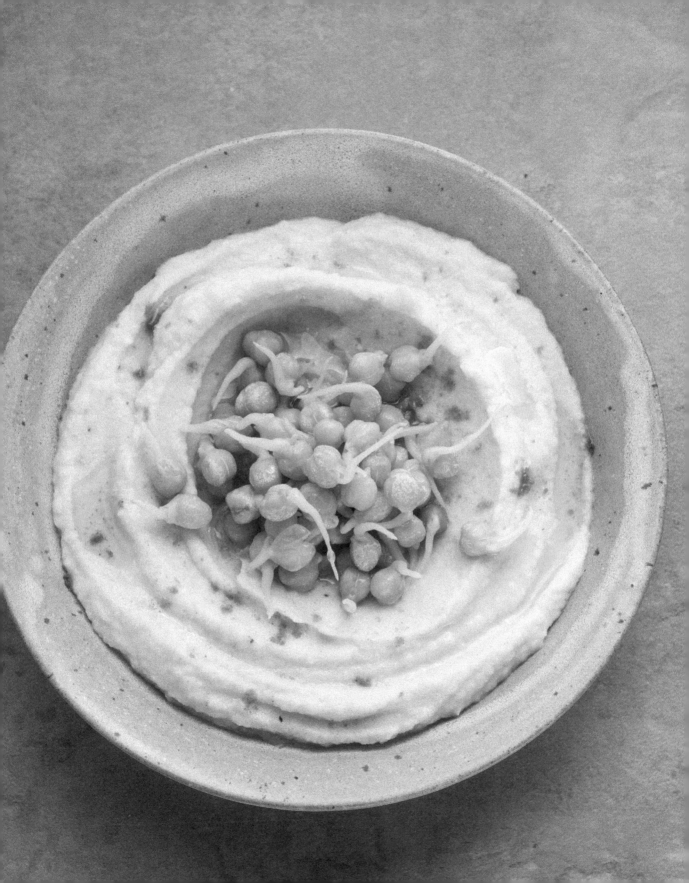

Red Pepper Pasta,
PAGE 86

VEGETARIAN MAINS

Lemon Tofu ■

PREP TIME: 10 MINUTES • **COOK TIME:** 25 MINUTES • **SERVES** 2

The lemon sauce in this recipe is well balanced with tart and sweet flavors. Inspired by something from the local Asian food court or restaurant, this has all the memories and taste without all the added salt.

½ cup dry parboiled white rice

1 tablespoon olive oil

2 medium green bell peppers, sliced

1 cup chopped bok choy

1 medium white onion, sliced

2 tablespoons lemon juice

¼ cup honey

½ cup vegetable broth, no added salt

6 ounces firm tofu, cut into ½-inch cubes

ADAPT FOR DIABETES:

Reduce the honey to 1 tablespoon and let the sauce simmer for a few minutes longer.

1. In a large pot, cook the rice according to the package directions, usually about 25 minutes. Drain and set aside.

2. Meanwhile, in a medium skillet over medium heat, heat the olive oil. Add the bell peppers, bok choy, and onion and stir-fry until the vegetables are tender but the peppers remain crisp. Set aside.

3. In the same pan, add the lemon juice, honey, and broth and let simmer for 10 minutes.

4. Add the tofu to the lemon sauce and stir to combine. Heat the tofu for about 5 minutes, until coated with the sauce. Serve with the vegetables and rice.

Per serving: Calories: 517; Protein: 15g; Total fat: 11g; Saturated fat: 1.5g; Total carbohydrates: 92g; Fiber: 5.5g; Cholesterol: 0mg; Phosphorus: 147mg; Potassium: 506mg; Sodium: 58mg; Sugar: 39g

Tofu Pad Thai ■

PREP TIME: 15 MINUTES • **COOK TIME:** 20 MINUTES • **SERVES** 4

Pad thai is a stir-fry dish with rice noodles, eggs, and tofu. It has a salty sweet-and-sour flavor, and while it's typically high in sodium, this option is low in sodium but loaded with flavor.

4 ounces dry rice noodles

2 cups Sweet-and-Sour Sauce (page 151)

2 limes, divided

3 tablespoons olive oil, divided

8 ounces firm tofu, sliced ½-inch thick

2 garlic cloves, minced

½ cup shredded carrots

1 cup snap peas

2 scallions, chopped, divided (white and green parts)

3 cups cabbage and carrot coleslaw mix

1 large egg

ADAPT FOR DIABETES:

Instead of rice noodles, use whole-grain spaghetti noodles and cook to al dente, or tender to the tooth.

---

1. Cook the noodles according to the package directions. Drain and set aside.

2. In a small bowl, combine the sauce and the juice of 1 lime. Set aside.

3. In a medium skillet, heat 1½ tablespoons of olive oil. Add the tofu and stir-fry until the tofu starts to brown, about 5 minutes. Transfer to a plate.

4. Add the remaining 1½ tablespoons of olive oil, the garlic, carrots, and snap peas to the skillet and stir-fry for about 30 seconds, until the vegetables are tender. Add the cooked noodles and 1 scallion, and stir-fry for a few seconds more.

5. Add the sauce to the skillet and stir to combine. Add the coleslaw mix and tofu. Stir-fry for about 3 minutes, until the noodles and vegetables are coated with the sauce. Transfer the noodle mix to a plate.

6. In the same skillet, scramble the egg until cooked. Then add the noodle mix back into the skillet and mix well. Transfer to a serving dish.

7. Garnish with the remaining scallion and the remaining lime, cut into wedges for squeezing.

Per serving: Calories: 408; Protein: 11g; Total fat: 14g; Saturated fat: 2g; Total carbohydrates: 63g; Fiber: 3.5g; Cholesterol: 46mg; Phosphorus: 56mg; Potassium: 231mg; Sodium: 176mg; Sugar: 31g

Minestrone ■

PREP TIME: 10 MINUTES • **COOK TIME:** 15 MINUTES • **SERVES** 4

Minestrone is an Italian vegetable soup that's thick and typically made from fresh vegetables like tomatoes, carrots, celery, and onion. This soup recipe is often called a kitchen-sink recipe because it includes vegetables that are on hand.

2 tablespoons olive oil

1 large white onion, diced

4 garlic cloves, minced

2 teaspoons dried parsley

2 teaspoons red pepper flakes

½ teaspoon freshly ground black pepper

4 cups vegetable broth, no added salt

1 (14.5-ounce) can diced tomatoes, no added salt

1 cup green beans, cut into ½-inch pieces

2 large carrots, cut into ½-inch rounds

½ cup diced celery

4 ounces dry orzo pasta

1. In a large pot over medium-low heat, heat the olive oil. Add the onion, garlic, parsley, red pepper flakes, and pepper. Cook until the onion softens, about 5 minutes.

2. Add the broth, tomatoes, green beans, carrots, and celery. Bring to a boil.

3. Add the pasta, bring the pot back to a simmer, and cook for about 5 minutes, or until the pasta is tender.

TIP: This soup is meant to be hearty and thick, so try adding additional vegetables like zucchini, spinach, or potatoes if potassium is not a concern.

Per serving: Calories: 253; Protein: 7g; Total fat: 7.5g; Saturated fat: 1g; Total carbohydrates: 39g; Fiber: 5.5g; Cholesterol: 0mg; Phosphorus: 43mg; Potassium: 500mg; Sodium: 79mg; Sugar: 9.5g

Carrot and Apple Soup ■

PREP TIME: 10 MINUTES • **COOK TIME:** 20 MINUTES • **SERVES** 4

This soup has gorgeous color and flavor combinations that are sure to give lots of warmth. Using staple ingredients like onion, carrots, and apples gives this soup loads of fiber, flavor, and fullness. This is an easy recipe to pull together, making it perfect for a weeknight meal.

1 tablespoon olive oil

1 small white onion, chopped

2 tablespoons chopped fresh ginger

4 large carrots, peeled and chopped

1 apple, peeled, cored, and chopped

8 ounces canned chickpeas, no added salt

3 teaspoons ground cinnamon

4 cups vegetable broth, no added salt

1½ cups unsweetened plain almond milk

1. In a large pot over medium heat, heat the olive oil. Add the onion and ginger. Cook until the onion is soft and translucent, about 5 minutes.

2. Add the carrots, apple, chickpeas, cinnamon, and broth.

3. Simmer the soup until the vegetables are tender, about 15 minutes.

4. Remove from the heat and pour the soup into a blender. Add the almond milk and blend until smooth. Alternatively, use an immersion blender, and blend the vegetables and almond milk in the pot until smooth.

TIP: Spice up this soup by adding 1 teaspoon turmeric and 1 teaspoon curry powder.

Per serving: Calories: 180; Protein: 5g; Total fat: 6g; Saturated fat: 0.5g; Total carbohydrates: 29g; Fiber: 8g; Cholesterol: 0mg; Phosphorus: 93mg; Potassium: 473mg; Sodium: 219mg; Sugar: 12g

Vegetarian Lasagna ■

PREP TIME: 15 MINUTES • **COOK TIME:** 50 MINUTES • **SERVES** 4

With layers of rich, roasted red pepper sauce, creamy cottage cheese filling, and fiber from savory vegetables, this lasagna is a crowd-pleaser. Serve it with a quick garden salad for a balanced meal.

1 tablespoon olive oil, divided

1 small white onion, minced

1 cup cubed eggplant

½ cup cubed zucchini

½ cup chopped green bell pepper

4 cups Roasted Red Pepper Sauce (page 149)

12 dry no-boil lasagna noodles

¾ cup low-fat smooth cottage cheese

½ cup shredded part-skim mozzarella cheese

ADAPT FOR HYPERTENSION:

Using a low-sodium tomato sauce is a great time-saver for this dish.

1. Preheat the oven to 375°F. Grease a loaf pan with ½ tablespoon of olive oil.

2. In a medium skillet over medium-high heat, heat the remaining ½ tablespoon of olive oil. Add the onion, eggplant, zucchini, and bell pepper and cook until the vegetables are soft, about 5 minutes.

3. Spread a thin layer of the pepper sauce on the bottom of the prepared pan. Then add a layer of noodles, followed by a layer of cottage cheese and vegetables, followed by another layer of noodles. Repeat until all the sauce, cottage cheese, and noodles are used. Top with the mozzarella and cover with aluminum foil.

4. Bake in the oven for 25 minutes. Remove the foil and bake for about an additional 20 minutes, or until the cheese is a golden brown.

TIP: Using homemade Roasted Red Pepper Sauce reduces the potassium content. If potassium is not an issue, substitute a no-added-salt tomato sauce.

Per serving: Calories: 627; Protein: 24g; Total fat: 16g; Saturated fat: 3.5g; Total carbohydrates: 94g; Fiber: 10g; Cholesterol: 11mg; Phosphorus: 282mg; Potassium: 716mg; Sodium: 659mg; Sugar: 17g

Mediterranean Eggplant Casserole ■

PREP TIME: 10 MINUTES • **COOK TIME:** 50 MINUTES • **SERVES** 4

The versatile eggplant comes in many colors and is a great source of fiber and antioxidants. This eggplant casserole has all the flavors of summer in one dish, but you can enjoy it all year long because it freezes well and is great for leftovers or weeknight dinners.

3 tablespoons olive oil, divided

1 large white onion, diced

2 garlic cloves, minced

1 medium green bell pepper, diced

1 cup canned diced tomatoes, no added salt

3 tablespoons dried parsley

1 tablespoon dried thyme

2 large eggplants, sliced into ½-inch pieces (8 cups)

1 tablespoon all-purpose flour

¼ cup shredded part-skim mozzarella cheese

ADAPT FOR CARDIOVASCULAR DISEASE:

Choose low-fat mozzarella cheese.

1. Preheat the oven to 375°F. Coat a casserole dish with 1½ tablespoons of olive oil.

2. In a large skillet, heat the remaining 1½ tablespoons of olive oil and sauté the onion until tender, about 10 minutes. Add the garlic and bell pepper and cook for about 3 minutes. Add the tomatoes, parsley, and thyme and simmer for a few minutes. Transfer the mixture to a bowl and set aside.

3. In the same skillet, add the eggplant, stirring frequently until browned, about 5 minutes. Add the flour and stir. Add the tomato mixture and bring to a simmer.

4. Spoon half of the vegetable mixture into the prepared casserole dish. Top with ⅛ cup of mozzarella cheese. Add the remaining vegetables and top with the remaining ⅛ cup of mozzarella cheese. Bake for about 30 minutes, or until the cheese is bubbly.

Per serving: Calories: 202; Protein: 5g; Total fat: 12g; Saturated fat: 2.5g; Total carbohydrates: 20g; Fiber: 6.5g; Cholesterol: 5mg; Phosphorus: 106mg; Potassium: 680mg; Sodium: 71mg; Sugar: 9.5g

Red Pepper Pasta ■

PREP TIME: 10 MINUTES · **COOK TIME:** 15 MINUTES · **SERVES** 4

Red peppers are a great source of vitamins A and C and antioxidants for over-all health. This pasta dish is a creamy, savory, and subtly sweet pasta, making it the perfect flavor companion for earthy mushrooms. This dish is easy to make and can be served warm or cold.

2 large red bell
  peppers, diced

½ cup halved white
  button mushrooms

2 tablespoons olive oil

2 garlic cloves, minced

8 ounces dry orzo pasta

2 cups Roasted Red
  Pepper Sauce (page 149)

4 tablespoons grated
  Parmesan cheese

1. Preheat the oven to 425°F. Line a baking sheet with parchment paper.

2. In a medium bowl, combine the bell peppers, mushrooms, olive oil, and garlic and toss together to coat with the olive oil. Transfer the vegetables to the prepared baking sheet and roast in the oven for about 15 minutes, or until soft.

3. Cook the pasta according to the package directions while the vegetables are roasting.

4. Drain and transfer the pasta to a large bowl. Coat the pasta with the pepper sauce, add the roasted vegetables, and combine. Top with the Parmesan cheese and serve warm.

TIP: Add 2 tablespoons of the pasta water to the pepper sauce for an extra-creamy sauce.

Per serving: Calories: 410; Protein: 11g; Total fat: 13g; Saturated fat: 2g; Total carbohydrates: 61g; Fiber: 6g; Cholesterol: 4mg; Phosphorus: 72mg; Potassium: 445mg; Sodium: 289mg; Sugar: 12g

Pineapple Fried Rice ■

PREP TIME: 15 MINUTES • **COOK TIME:** 30 MINUTES • **SERVES** 2

This meal comes together in a snap and combines sweet pineapple, garlic, and soy sauce to create a comforting and satisfying meal. This recipe is also a great way to use leftover rice, which will save more time.

½ cup dry parboiled rice

2 tablespoons olive oil, divided

2 (8-ounce) cans juice-packed pineapple chunks, drained

1 large green bell pepper, diced

2 scallions, chopped (white and green parts)

2 garlic cloves, minced

2 large eggs, beaten

1 tablespoon reduced-sodium soy sauce

2 tablespoons lime juice

ADAPT FOR DIABETES:

Try making this recipe with whole-grain rice for more fiber.

1. Cook the rice according to the package directions, usually about 25 minutes. Drain and set aside to cool.

2. Heat 1 tablespoon of oil in a medium skillet over medium heat. Add the pineapple and bell pepper. Cook for about 3 minutes. Add the scallions and garlic and cook until fragrant, about 30 seconds. Set aside.

3. In a large skillet, heat the remaining 1 tablespoon of oil. Add the eggs and cook, stirring frequently, until the eggs are scrambled.

4. Add the rice and vegetables to the eggs in the pan. Add the soy sauce and lime juice, stirring to coat. Serve immediately.

Per serving: Calories: 519; Protein: 13g; Total fat: 19g; Saturated fat: 3.5g; Total carbohydrates: 76g; Fiber: 5g; Cholesterol: 186mg; Phosphorus: 215mg; Potassium: 586mg; Sodium: 368mg; Sugar: 29g

Grilled Paneer Sandwich ■

PREP TIME: 15 MINUTES • **COOK TIME:** 10 MINUTES • **SERVES 4**

Paneer is a fresh, non-melting soft cheese, often used in Indian cuisine. Marinating the creamy texture of paneer in the flavorful Roasted Red Pepper sauce makes a delicious twist on a grilled cheese sandwich. Paneer is a great protein and a source of calcium to keep bones and teeth strong.

3 ounces paneer, sliced

1 cup Roasted Red Pepper Sauce (page 149), divided

2 tablespoons unsalted butter

8 small slices sourdough bread

2 portobello mushrooms, sliced

1 medium green bell pepper, thinly sliced

½ small red onion, thinly sliced

1. Marinate the paneer slices in ½ cup of pepper sauce for 10 minutes.

2. Spread ½ tablespoon of butter evenly over one side of each slice of bread.

3. Heat a large skillet over medium heat.

4. Lay four slices of bread, butter-side down, in the skillet. Top each slice with ⅛ cup of the remaining pepper sauce. Next, layer even portions of the marinated paneer, mushrooms, bell pepper, and onion. Top with the remaining slices of bread, butter-side up, to make 4 sandwiches.

5. After 1 to 2 minutes, flip the sandwiches. Continue to flip the sandwiches until both sides of the bread are golden brown. This recipe can also be prepared in a sandwich press.

TIME-SAVING TIP: Swap the homemade sauce for a low-sodium pesto sauce.

TIP: If paneer cheese is not available, low-fat mozzarella makes a great gooey alternative.

Per serving: Calories: 356; Protein: 13g; Total fat: 14g; Saturated fat: 7.5g; Total carbohydrates: 44g; Fiber: 4g; Cholesterol: 34mg; Phosphorus: 125mg; Potassium: 398mg; Sodium: 492mg; Sugar: 9g

Chickpea Curry ■

PREP TIME: 10 MINUTES • **COOK TIME:** 30 MINUTES • **SERVES** 4

Chickpeas are a legume packed with protein and fiber. The aroma and flavors in this recipe will appeal to the senses as the chickpeas take on the flavors of the herbs and spices, making a comfy and cozy dish. This curry is wonderful served over rice or with naan and a salad.

2 tablespoons olive oil

2 medium white onions, 1 chopped and 1 grated

4 garlic cloves, minced

1 tablespoon finely chopped fresh ginger

¼ teaspoon freshly ground black pepper

1 teaspoon ground cumin

2 teaspoons ground cinnamon

1 (15-ounce) can chickpeas, no added salt, drained and rinsed

1½ cups water

2 tablespoons lemon juice

ADAPT FOR DIABETES:

Use parboiled rice for a low-glycemic-index option.

1. In a large pot over medium heat, heat the olive oil. Add the chopped onion and cook until the onion is lightly golden, about 5 minutes.

2. Add the grated onion, garlic, ginger, and pepper. Cook for about 2 minutes, or until fragrant.

3. Add the cumin and cinnamon and heat for about 5 minutes. Stir while heating.

4. Mash 1 cup of chickpeas, using a potato masher or fork. Add the mashed and remaining whole chickpeas to the pot. Stir to mix evenly.

5. Add the water and lemon juice and stir. Let simmer for 10 minutes, covered.

6. Serve warm.

Per serving: Calories: 185; Protein: 6g; Total fat: 8.5g; Saturated fat: 1g; Total carbohydrates: 23g; Fiber: 6.5g; Cholesterol: 0mg; Phosphorus: 103mg; Potassium: 284mg; Sodium: 124mg; Sugar: 6.5g

Peanut-Chili Tofu with Noodles ■

PREP TIME: 10 MINUTES • **COOK TIME:** 20 MINUTES • **SERVES** 2

Full of sesame and peanut butter flavors, this meal is sure to make the mouth water. It tastes great warm or cold, so be sure to try it both ways.

4 ounces dry spaghetti

2 tablespoons unsalted peanut butter

1 tablespoon sesame oil

1 tablespoon rice vinegar

2 garlic cloves, minced

1 tablespoon minced fresh ginger

1 tablespoon olive oil

1 small red onion, chopped

1 medium green bell pepper, sliced

1 cup grated carrots

6 ounces firm tofu, cut into cubes

ADAPT FOR DIABETES:

Cook the pasta to al dente for a lower-glycemic-index option.

1. Cook the spaghetti according to the package directions. Drain and set aside.

2. In a small bowl, mix the peanut butter, sesame oil, rice vinegar, garlic, and ginger. Set aside.

3. In a medium pan over medium heat, heat the olive oil. Add the onion, bell pepper, and carrots and cook until soft, about 5 minutes.

4. Add the tofu to the pan with the vegetables and cook until soft, about 5 minutes.

5. In the same pan, coat the tofu and vegetables with an ⅛ cup of peanut butter sauce.

6. Add the spaghetti noodles and the remaining ⅛ cup of sauce to the tofu and vegetables. Coat and mix everything well.

TIP: Top with red pepper flakes for added heat.

Per serving: Calories: 557; Protein: 20g; Total fat: 26g; Saturated fat: 4g; Total carbohydrates: 62g; Fiber: 6.5g; Cholesterol: 0mg; Phosphorus: 208mg; Potassium: 571mg; Sodium: 163mg; Sugar: 11g

Chickpea Bolognese ■

PREP TIME: 10 MINUTES • **COOK TIME:** 20 MINUTES • **SERVES** 4

This quick-and-easy plant-based dish has a deep flavorful sauce that is hearty and packed with protein and fiber from the chickpeas. Using canned chickpeas helps cut down on the time in the kitchen. Chopping the chickpeas makes them easier to eat with noodles.

8 ounces dry spaghetti pasta

1 tablespoon olive oil

1 medium white onion, chopped

3 garlic cloves, minced

½ cup shredded carrots

1 (14.5-ounce) can diced tomatoes, no added salt

3 teaspoons dried parsley

1 teaspoon red pepper flakes

1 cup canned chickpeas, no added salt, drained and chopped

4 tablespoons grated Parmesan cheese

ADAPT FOR HYPERTENSION:

Reduce the portion of Parmesan cheese in order to lower the sodium in this meal.

1. Cook the pasta according to the package directions. Drain and set aside.

2. In a separate pot over medium heat, heat the olive oil. Add the onion, garlic, and carrots. Cook until the vegetables are tender, about 5 minutes.

3. Add the tomatoes, parsley, and red pepper flakes to the pot. Stir and let simmer for 5 minutes.

4. Add the chickpeas to the sauce and simmer for 10 minutes.

5. Serve the pasta sauce over the noodles garnished with the Parmesan cheese.

TIP: This recipe is also great with no-salt-added canned lentils.

Per serving: Calories: 358; Protein: 13g; Total fat: 7g; Saturated fat: 1.5g; Total carbohydrates: 60g; Fiber: 6g; Cholesterol: 4mg; Phosphorus: 201mg; Potassium: 512mg; Sodium: 201mg; Sugar: 7g

Sweet and Spicy Tofu Stir-Fry ■

PREP TIME: 20 MINUTES • **COOK TIME:** 20 MINUTES • **SERVES** 4

Tofu is a great kitchen staple to have handy because it's full of protein. In this recipe, tofu takes on the flavors of this sweet and spicy marinade while also being a great source of protein for kidney, heart, and diabetes health.

1½ cups dry parboiled rice

14 ounces firm tofu, cut into cubes

1 cup sliced yellow onion

½ cup sliced carrot

1 cup sliced green bell pepper

1 cup broccoli florets

½ cup sliced white button mushrooms

2 cups Stir-Fry Sauce (page 148)

2 tablespoons honey

2 teaspoons red pepper flakes

1. Cook the rice according to the package directions. Drain and set aside.

2. In a wok or medium skillet over medium-high heat, cook the tofu, onion, carrot, bell pepper, broccoli, and mushrooms for about 10 minutes, or until crisp-tender.

3. In a small bowl, combine the sauce, honey, and pepper flakes and pour over the tofu and vegetable mixture. Simmer for 5 minutes on medium-high heat to thicken the sauce.

4. Serve the tofu and vegetable stir-fry with rice.

TIP: For a time-saving swap, replace the fry sauce with a reduced-sodium soy sauce (2 tablespoons) and flavor with sesame oil (2 teaspoons).

Per serving: Calories: 493; Protein: 20g; Total fat: 5.5g; Saturated fat: 1g; Total carbohydrates: 92g; Fiber: 5g; Cholesterol: 0mg; Phosphorus: 208mg; Potassium: 540mg; Sodium: 989mg; Sugar: 26g

Black Bean Enchiladas ■

PREP TIME: 15 MINUTES • **COOK TIME:** 50 MINUTES • **SERVES** 4

Filled with black beans, colorful vegetables, and a secret low-sodium enchilada sauce, these enchiladas are a hearty entrée. These enchiladas can be prepared with either corn or flour tortillas and are best served with a side salad to balance the meal.

3 tablespoons olive oil, divided

1 small white onion, chopped

1 medium green bell pepper, chopped

1 teaspoon ground cumin

½ teaspoon ground cinnamon

1 (14-ounce) can black beans, no added salt, drained and rinsed

½ cup shredded part-skim mozzarella cheese, divided

2 cups Enchilada Sauce (page 150), divided

4 Homemade Flour Tortillas (page 147)

1. Preheat the oven to 400°F. Coat a casserole dish with 1 tablespoon of olive oil.

2. In a large skillet over medium-high heat, heat the remaining 2 tablespoons of olive oil. Add the onion and bell pepper and cook, stirring occasionally, until tender, about 10 minutes.

3. Add the cumin and cinnamon to the vegetables and stir. Add the beans, ¼ cup of cheese, and 2 tablespoons of enchilada sauce and stir to combine.

4. Coat the bottom of the prepared casserole dish with ¼ cup of enchilada sauce and assemble the enchiladas by spooning ½ cup of the bean and cheese mixture into the middle of a tortilla and folding the edges over to make a wrap. Place seam-side down in the casserole dish. Repeat with the remaining tortillas.

5. Cover the enchiladas with the remaining 1¾ cups of sauce and ¼ cup of cheese. Bake uncovered for about 20 minutes, or until the cheese is golden brown.

Per serving: Calories: 423; Protein: 15g; Total fat: 18g; Saturated fat: 3.5g; Total carbohydrates: 51g; Fiber: 8.5g; Cholesterol: 9mg; Phosphorus: 224mg; Potassium: 468mg; Sodium: 329mg; Sugar: 3.5g

Lemon-Garlic Mussels,
PAGE 105

CHAPTER 6

SEAFOOD

Mediterranean Cod ■

PREP TIME: 10 MINUTES • **COOK TIME:** 20 MINUTES • **SERVES** 4

This easy-to-make and colorful Mediterranean-inspired cod is packed with flavor from the tomatoes, leeks, parsley, and garlic. The leeks in this recipe offer an aroma similar to the onion but have additional fiber and are also a low-potassium vegetable.

8 ounces skinless fresh cod

1 medium green bell pepper, quartered

2 Roma tomatoes, quartered

1 medium white onion, quartered

4 leeks, chopped (white and light green parts)

2 tablespoons olive oil

1 teaspoon freshly ground black pepper

1 teaspoon red pepper flakes

1 teaspoon dried parsley

1 teaspoon garlic powder

ADAPT FOR CKD STAGE 5:

Double the cod in this recipe for a high-protein option.

1. Preheat the oven to 425°F. Line a baking sheet with parchment paper.

2. Place the cod on the prepared baking sheet and arrange the bell pepper, tomatoes, onion, and leeks around it.

3. In a small bowl, combine the olive oil, pepper, red pepper flakes, parsley, and garlic powder. Drizzle over the fish and vegetables on the baking sheet.

4. Bake in the oven for about 20 minutes, or until the fish is flaky, tender, and no longer translucent.

Per serving: Calories: 183; Protein: 11g; Total fat: 7.5g; Saturated fat: 1g; Total carbohydrates: 19g; Fiber: 3.5g; Cholesterol: 22mg; Phosphorus: 112mg; Potassium: 451mg; Sodium: 53mg; Sugar: 6g

Grilled Cod with Pineapple Salsa ■

PREP TIME: 10 MINUTES • **COOK TIME:** 10 MINUTES • **SERVES** 4

Cod is a great kidney-friendly protein because, compared to other whitefish options, it is lower in potassium and phosphorus. The pineapple salsa in this recipe is a refreshing condiment that will bring a pop of color to this meal. The pineapple has antioxidants and a digestive enzyme called bromelain to help break down proteins in the fish.

2 (8-ounce) cans juice-packed pineapple chunks

½ cup chopped green bell pepper

¼ cup chopped cherry tomatoes

¼ cup chopped red onion

1 small jalapeño, seeded and chopped

2 tablespoons lime juice

3 teaspoons dried parsley

¼ cup all-purpose flour

1 teaspoon freshly ground black pepper

1 teaspoon chili powder

8 ounces skinless fresh cod

1 tablespoon olive oil

1. In a medium bowl, mix the pineapple, bell pepper, tomatoes, onion, jalapeño, lime juice, and parsley. Store in the refrigerator until ready to serve.

2. Place the flour, pepper, and chili powder on a large plate and combine. Coat the fish in the flour mixture.

3. In a medium skillet over medium-high heat, heat the olive oil. Add the fish and cook for 3 to 4 minutes per side until tender, flaky, and no longer translucent inside.

4. Serve the fish with the pineapple salsa.

Per serving: Calories: 161; Protein: 11g; Total fat: 4g; Saturated fat: 0.5g; Total carbohydrates: 22g; Fiber: 2g; Cholesterol: 22mg; Phosphorus: 77mg; Potassium: 347mg; Sodium: 39mg; Sugar: 14g

Lemon-Butter Tilapia ■

PREP TIME: 5 MINUTES • **COOK TIME:** 15 MINUTES • **SERVES** 4

The cooked fish is tender and melts in the mouth. It is best enjoyed immediately but can easily be used as leftovers. Tilapia, a great budget-friendly fish, is quick to prepare so it can be enjoyed during the weeknight hustle.

1 teaspoon freshly ground black pepper

3 tablespoons unsalted butter, melted

1 tablespoon garlic powder

½ teaspoon red pepper flakes

½ teaspoon dried parsley

2 tablespoons lemon juice

8 ounces fresh tilapia

1 lemon, sliced into rounds

ADAPT FOR CARDIOVASCULAR DISEASE:

Replace the butter with plant-sterol-enriched margarine.

1. Preheat the oven to 400°F. Line a baking sheet with parchment paper.

2. In a medium bowl, mix the pepper, butter, garlic powder, red pepper flakes, parsley, and lemon juice.

3. Place the tilapia on the prepared baking sheet and pour the lemon-butter mixture over the fish to coat. Top with the lemon slices.

4. Bake in the oven for 10 to 12 minutes, until the fish is tender and flaky.

TIP: This recipe can also be made with other kidney-friendly fish such as sole, cod, or salmon.

Per serving: Calories: 143; Protein: 12g; Total fat: 9.5g; Saturated fat: 5.5g; Total carbohydrates: 3g; Fiber: 0.5g; Cholesterol: 51mg; Phosphorus: 111mg; Potassium: 223mg; Sodium: 33mg; Sugar: 0g

Spicy Ginger Tilapia Soup ■

PREP TIME: 5 MINUTES • **COOK TIME:** 15 MINUTES • **SERVES** 4

This refreshing soup is great for a light meal but still packs a lot of flavor. The fish in this soup takes on the seasonings of the red pepper flakes and fresh ginger, which balance out the lime. This is a complete meal in a bowl.

1 tablespoon olive oil

3 tablespoons minced fresh ginger

1 cup chopped scallions (white and green parts)

3 garlic cloves, chopped

1 cup snap peas

1 medium green bell pepper, sliced

4 cups water

6 ounces fresh tilapia

2 tablespoons lime juice

1 tablespoon red pepper flakes

1. In a large pot over medium heat, heat the olive oil. Add the ginger, scallions, and garlic and sauté until fragrant, about 3 minutes.

2. Add the snap peas and bell pepper and cook for about 5 minutes, or until tender.

3. Add the water and fish and bring to a boil. Lower the temperature to low and simmer the fish thoroughly for about 10 minutes, or until the fish is flaky and tender and no longer translucent.

4. Add the lime juice and red pepper flakes and stir. Enjoy.

TIP: Replace the water with no-added-salt vegetable broth for a richer flavor.

Per serving: Calories: 111; Protein: 10g; Total fat: 4.5g; Saturated fat: 1g; Total carbohydrates: 8g; Fiber: 2.5g; Cholesterol: 21mg; Phosphorus: 97mg; Potassium: 313mg; Sodium: 29mg; Sugar: 3g

Shrimp Spaghetti ■

PREP TIME: 10 MINUTES • **COOK TIME:** 20 MINUTES • **SERVES** 4

This easy-to-prepare meal is a kidney-friendly spin on a classic Italian dish. The aroma from the garlic and onions is incredibly inviting and satisfying to the taste buds. Serve either warm or cold.

8 ounces dry spaghetti pasta

1 tablespoon olive oil

1 medium white onion, chopped

4 garlic cloves, minced

1 medium green bell pepper, chopped

½ pound shrimp, peeled and deveined

1 teaspoon red pepper flakes

1 teaspoon freshly ground black pepper

½ cup chicken broth, no added salt

2 tablespoons lemon juice

1 tablespoon lemon zest

2 tablespoons dried parsley

ADAPT FOR CKD STAGE 5:

Add an extra ¼ pound of shrimp or low-sodium canned oysters for a high-protein option.

1. Cook the pasta according to the package directions. Drain and set aside.

2. While the pasta is boiling, in a large skillet over medium-high heat, heat the olive oil. Add the onion, garlic, and bell pepper and sauté for about 2 minutes, or until the onion is translucent. Add the shrimp, red pepper flakes, and pepper. Cook the shrimp for about 5 minutes, or until pink.

3. Add the broth, lemon juice, lemon zest, and parsley, mixing to combine. Let the sauce boil down for about 5 minutes, or until reduced by half. Toss with the pasta and serve.

Per serving: Calories: 251; Protein: 25g; Total fat: 4.5g; Saturated fat: 1g; Total carbohydrates: 28g; Fiber: 2.5g; Cholesterol: 160mg; Phosphorus: 290mg; Potassium: 475mg; Sodium: 134mg; Sugar: 3g

Shrimp Fried Rice ∎

PREP TIME: 15 MINUTES • **COOK TIME:** 20 MINUTES • **SERVES** 4

This shrimp fried rice is better than takeout on so many levels. It is packed with flavor, lacks all the grease typically found with fried rice, and is a lower-sodium option. The twist on this fried rice is the addition of vegetables for extra fiber and fullness.

1 cup dry parboiled rice

1 tablespoon olive oil

1 large egg

¼ pound shrimp, peeled and deveined

1 teaspoon sesame oil

1 medium green bell pepper, chopped

1 medium white onion, chopped

2 cups shredded carrots

2 cups chopped broccoli

¼ cup reduced-sodium soy sauce

1 teaspoon red pepper flakes

1. Cook the rice according to the package directions. Drain and set aside.

2. In a medium skillet over medium heat, heat the olive oil. Add the egg and scramble for about 2 minutes, or until it reaches your desired doneness. Remove the egg and set aside.

3. Add the shrimp to the pan and cook for 2 to 3 minutes per side. Remove the shrimp and set aside.

4. In the same pan, heat the sesame oil. Add the bell pepper, onion, carrots, and broccoli and sauté for 10 minutes, or until the vegetables are al dente.

5. Combine the shrimp, rice, and eggs in the pan with the vegetables. Add the soy sauce and red pepper flakes. Stir to combine well. Serve immediately.

Per serving: Calories: 306; Protein: 14g; Total fat: 6.5g; Saturated fat: 1g; Total carbohydrates: 49g; Fiber: 4g; Cholesterol: 86mg; Phosphorus: 219mg; Potassium: 460mg; Sodium: 660mg; Sugar: 4.5g

Honey, Lime, and Garlic Baked Salmon ■

PREP TIME: 5 MINUTES • **COOK TIME:** 20 MINUTES • **SERVES** 4

This tender and flavorful meal comes with a hint of lime and can be eaten hot or cold. This salmon would be great with vegetables, salad, or Garlic Double-Boiled Potatoes (page 66). Packed with flavor, this nutrient-dense meal provides omega-3s, antioxidants, and fiber, all of which are important for kidney health.

⅛ cup honey

2 garlic cloves, minced

2 tablespoons lime juice

1 teaspoon freshly ground black pepper

½ teaspoon red pepper flakes

8 ounces fresh salmon

1 lime, sliced

ADAPT FOR CKD STAGE 5:

For a high-protein option, double the recipe.

1. Preheat the oven to 400°F. Line a baking sheet with parchment paper.

2. In a small bowl, combine the honey, garlic, lime juice, pepper, and red pepper flakes.

3. Place the salmon on the prepared baking sheet and coat with the sauce. Top the fish with the lime slices.

4. Bake for 12 to 15 minutes, until the fish is tender and flaky. Adjust the oven to broil and broil the fish for an additional 3 minutes.

TIP: Add lime zest after cooking for a double hit of citrus and a tangy finish.

Per serving: Calories: 130; Protein: 13g; Total fat: 4g; Saturated fat: 0.5g; Total carbohydrates: 10g; Fiber: 0.5g; Cholesterol: 36mg; Phosphorus: 135mg; Potassium: 349mg; Sodium: 29mg; Sugar: 8g

Spicy Salmon ■

PREP TIME: 5 MINUTES • **COOK TIME:** 20 MINUTES • **SERVES** 4

This easy recipe will turn anyone into a salmon lover. With sweet, salty, and spicy notes, the idea that this is a nutritious and low-sodium meal will be forgotten immediately. Leftovers may be refrigerated in an airtight container for 2 days. To help with the fishy smell while storing, flake the salmon before putting it in the refrigerator.

4 garlic cloves, minced

¼ cup reduced-sodium soy sauce

1 tablespoon honey

1 tablespoon red pepper flakes

8 ounces salmon, skin on

ADAPT FOR HYPERTENSION:

Reduce the soy sauce by half and add 2 teaspoons sesame oil for extra flavor.

1. Preheat the oven to 400°F. Line a baking sheet with parchment paper or use a cast-iron grill pan.

2. In a small bowl, mix the garlic, soy sauce, honey, and red pepper flakes. Coat the meat side of the fish with the mixture.

3. Place the coated fish, skin-side down, on the prepared baking sheet or grill pan. Bake in the oven for 15 to 20 minutes, until the salmon is flaky. Serve immediately.

Per serving: Calories: 126; Protein: 15g; Total fat: 4.5g; Saturated fat: 0.5g; Total carbohydrates: 7g; Fiber: 0.5g; Cholesterol: 36mg; Phosphorus: 165mg; Potassium: 415mg; Sodium: 605mg; Sugar: 4g

Crab Salad ■

PREP TIME: 10 MINUTES • **SERVES** 4

Crab is a lean shellfish low in potassium and phosphorus, making it a great source of protein for a kidney-friendly diet. This crab salad is refreshing with bits of lemon and pepper and is great served with a salad on a summer day.

4 ounces canned
low-sodium crabmeat

3 tablespoons lemon juice

3 tablespoons olive
oil, divided

2 tablespoons
dried parsley

½ teaspoon freshly
ground black pepper

8 cups arugula

1 small red bell
pepper, sliced

4 small slices
sourdough bread

1. In a medium bowl, toss together the crabmeat, lemon juice, 1½ tablespoons of olive oil, the parsley, and pepper.

2. In a separate medium bowl, toss the arugula, bell pepper, and remaining 1½ tablespoon of olive oil together.

3. Divide the arugula among the salad bowls and top each with an even amount of the crab mixture. Serve with the sourdough bread.

Per serving: Calories: 228; Protein: 10g; Total fat: 11g; Saturated fat: 1.5g; Total carbohydrates: 22g; Fiber: 2.5g; Cholesterol: 30mg; Phosphorus: 43mg; Potassium: 115mg; Sodium: 354mg; Sugar: 4.5g

Lemon-Garlic Mussels ■

PREP TIME: 10 MINUTES • **COOK TIME:** 20 MINUTES • **SERVES** 4

Mussels are an often-underappreciated shellfish, but they are a great source of heart-healthy omega-3s. The bread-soaking sauce is loaded with buttery garlic (without real butter) and lemon flavors that will make any mouth water. Garnish with fresh parsley for a pop of color.

2 tablespoons olive oil

4 garlic cloves, minced

1 small white onion, chopped

1 pound raw mussels

2 tablespoons lemon juice

3 tablespoons dried parsley

1 teaspoon freshly ground black pepper

ADAPT FOR CKD STAGE 5:

Add an extra ½ pound of mussels because they are a great protein and omega-3 source.

1. In a medium skillet with a lid over medium-high heat, heat the olive oil. Add the garlic and onion and sauté for 2 minutes, or until fragrant.

2. Add the mussels to the skillet and toss. Cover the pan, lower the heat to medium-low, and cook the mussels for 10 to 15 minutes, until the mussels open. Discard any unopened mussels.

3. Uncover the skillet and add the lemon juice, parsley, and pepper and toss together. Serve immediately.

TIP: Mussels are alive until just before cooking. Be sure to practice good food safety when preparing.

Per serving: Calories: 175; Protein: 14g; Total fat: 9.5g; Saturated fat: 1.5g; Total carbohydrates: 8g; Fiber: 1g; Cholesterol: 32mg; Phosphorus: 239mg; Potassium: 446mg; Sodium: 331mg; Sugar: 1g

Spicy Panfried Tilapia ■

PREP TIME: 5 MINUTES • **COOK TIME:** 10 MINUTES • **SERVES** 4

The hint of lime in this dish takes the Caribbean seasoning to the next level by adding a fresh citrus flavor that balances out the spice. A quick-and-easy recipe that can be made for a weeknight dinner or entertaining guests, the flavors will not disappoint.

8 ounces fresh tilapia

2½ tablespoons Caribbean Seasoning Mix (page 152)

2 tablespoons olive oil

2 tablespoons lime juice

ADAPT FOR CKD STAGE 5:

Increase the tilapia portion by 2 ounces.

1. Coat the fish with the seasoning mix.

2. In a medium skillet over medium-high heat, heat the olive oil. Add the fish and sauté for 3 to 4 minutes per side, until flaky and no longer translucent.

3. Season with the lime juice before removing from the pan. Serve immediately.

TIP: Try serving this recipe with grilled pineapple slices for a refreshing side dish.

Per serving: Calories: 129; Protein: 12g; Total fat: 8g; Saturated fat: 1g; Total carbohydrates: 3.5g; Fiber: 1g; Cholesterol: 28mg; Phosphorus: 110mg; Potassium: 231mg; Sodium: 39mg; Sugar: 0.5g

Sheet Pan Cod and Roasted Vegetables ■

PREP TIME: 10 MINUTES • **COOK TIME:** 20 MINUTES • **SERVES** 4

Sheet pan meals make cooking and cleanup quick and simple. The fresh vegetables in this recipe can last a long time in the refrigerator, so this recipe can be enjoyed any time of the week. These vegetables are also great sources of vitamin C and antioxidants, and they help the body maintain homeostasis from the acid-base balance.

3 tablespoons olive oil

3 tablespoons lemon juice, plus additional for drizzling

1 tablespoon dried parsley

2 teaspoons freshly ground black pepper

3 cups green beans

1 medium green bell pepper, sliced

2 cups cauliflower, chopped

12 ounces skinless fresh cod

1. Preheat the oven to 425°F. Line a baking sheet with parchment paper.

2. In a medium bowl, mix the olive oil, lemon juice, parsley, and pepper to create a marinade. Add the green beans and bell pepper and mix. Place the vegetables on the bottom third of the prepared baking sheet, reserving the leftover marinade in the bowl.

3. Toss the cauliflower in the leftover marinade and place on the middle third the of the baking sheet. Again, reserve the leftover marinade in the bowl.

4. Place the fish on the top third of the baking sheet and drizzle with the remaining marinade.

5. Roast for about 20 minutes, or until the fish is flaky and tender. Season with additional lemon juice before serving.

Per serving: Calories: 187; Protein: 16g; Total fat: 11g; Saturated fat: 1.5g; Total carbohydrates: 8g; Fiber: 3g; Cholesterol: 32mg; Phosphorus: 128mg; Potassium: 450mg; Sodium: 67mg; Sugar: 3g

Caribbean Cod Tacos ■

PREP TIME: 20 MINUTES • **COOK TIME:** 10 MINUTES • **SERVES** 4

This meal comes together in less than 30 minutes and is filled with spicy and sweet flavors. The word taco means "light lunch," but there really isn't a right or wrong time to eat a taco. These tacos may make for messy hands, so do have a napkin handy.

2 cups shredded green cabbage

1 cup shredded red cabbage

1 cup shredded carrots

2 scallions, chopped (white and green parts)

½ cup canned juice-packed pineapple chunks

1 tablespoon honey

2½ tablespoons olive oil, divided

2 tablespoons lime juice

8 ounces skinless fresh cod

2½ tablespoons Caribbean Seasoning Mix (page 152)

8 Homemade Flour Tortillas (page 147)

ADAPT FOR DIABETES:

Choose canned pineapple in water instead of simple syrup or juice.

1. In a medium bowl, combine the green cabbage, red cabbage, carrots, scallions, and pineapple chunks.

2. In a separate bowl, whisk together the honey, 2 tablespoons of olive oil, and the lime juice. Coat the cabbage mixture with the marinade and set aside.

3. Coat the fish with the Caribbean seasoning.

4. Heat a medium skillet over medium heat. Coat the pan with the remaining ½ tablespoon of olive oil. Add seasoned fish to the pan and cook 3 to 4 minutes per side, until flaky.

5. Serve the fish and coleslaw in the tortillas as a fish taco.

Per serving: Calories: 475; Protein: 17g; Total fat: 16g; Saturated fat: 2.5g; Total carbohydrates: 66g; Fiber: 4.5g; Cholesterol: 22mg; Phosphorus: 154mg; Potassium: 385mg; Sodium: 354mg; Sugar: 12g

Lemon Salmon Patties ■

PREP TIME: 15 MINUTES • **COOK TIME:** 10 MINUTES • **SERVES** 4

Salmon patties are similar to a fish cake. These homemade patties are moist, flavorful, and versatile, and they use old-fashioned rolled oats for extra fiber. Enjoy them with a salad for a quick, budget-friendly, and kidney-friendly meal. These patties go well with a salad or atop brioche buns.

1 (8-ounce) can skinless, boneless salmon

1 small white onion, chopped

1 celery stalk, chopped

2 tablespoons dried parsley

1 large egg

½ cup old-fashioned rolled oats

1 tablespoon olive oil

Rosemary-Garlic Sauce (page 154)

ADAPT FOR HYPERTENSION:

Choose canned salmon in water.

1. In a medium bowl, combine the salmon, onion, celery, parsley, egg, and oats. Form into four even patties.

2. In a medium skillet over medium heat, heat the olive oil and place the patties evenly spaced in the skillet. Cook until golden brown, about 5 minutes, then flip to cook the other side, about 5 minutes more.

3. Serve the salmon patties topped with the Rosemary-Garlic Sauce.

TIP: Use canned tuna for a milder taste.

Per serving: Calories: 180; Protein: 13g; Total fat: 9.5g; Saturated fat: 3g; Total carbohydrates: 11g; Fiber: 2g; Cholesterol: 77mg; Phosphorus: 75mg; Potassium: 139mg; Sodium: 240mg; Sugar: 2g

Garlic Shrimp Pasta ■

PREP TIME: 10 MINUTES • **COOK TIME:** 20 MINUTES • **SERVES** 4

This is an easy weeknight pasta dish that can be whipped up in 30 minutes or less. This dish is simple, flavorful, and satisfying as a classic comfort meal for summer or winter.

8 ounces dry
spaghetti pasta

2 tablespoons olive oil

1 medium white
onion, chopped

4 garlic cloves, minced

12 cherry tomatoes

1 pound shrimp, peeled
and deveined

2 teaspoons red
pepper flakes

¾ cup chicken broth, no
added salt

1 teaspoon freshly ground
black pepper

1 teaspoon dried parsley

**ADAPT FOR CKD
STAGES 1 TO 4:**

*Reduce the shrimp to
½ pound and add a
sliced bell pepper for a
lower-protein option.*

1. Cook the pasta according to the package directions. Drain and set aside.

2. Meanwhile, in a medium skillet over medium heat, heat the olive oil. Add the onion and garlic and sauté until tender, about 5 minutes.

3. Add the tomatoes, shrimp, and red pepper flakes and cook for 5 minutes, or until the shrimp start to turn pink.

4. Add the broth and pepper to the shrimp and let cook for 2 to 4 minutes, until the shrimp are pink and cooked thorough.

5. Remove the skillet from the heat, add the pasta and parsley to the shrimp, and toss to mix. Serve immediately.

Per serving: Calories: 388; Protein: 29g; Total fat: 8.5g; Saturated fat: 1g; Total carbohydrates: 49g; Fiber: 3.5g; Cholesterol: 160mg; Phosphorus: 347mg; Potassium: 586mg; Sodium: 139mg; Sugar: 4g

Shrimp Stir-Fry ■

PREP TIME: 15 MINUTES • **COOK TIME:** 20 MINUTES • **SERVES** 4

Including sesame oil at the end of this recipe adds a luscious nutty flavor note to the stir-fry. Made from sesame seeds, sesame oil does not turn rancid or develop a bad flavor when cooked at high temperatures, making it a great addition to stir-fry meals. Sesame oil is also a great source of omega-3s for cardiovascular health.

1 tablespoon olive oil

2 cups broccoli florets

1 medium green bell pepper, chopped

1 medium white onion, chopped

1 cup sugar snap peas

1 pound medium shrimp, peeled and deveined

1 cup Stir-Fry Sauce (page 148)

2 teaspoons sesame oil

2 cups cooked parboiled white rice

1. In a medium skillet over medium-high heat, heat the olive oil. Add the broccoli, bell pepper, onion, and snap peas. Cook until tender, about 10 minutes.

2. Add the shrimp to the vegetable mixture in the skillet and cook for 2 to 3 minutes per side.

3. Add the sauce and coat the shrimp and vegetables. Add the sesame oil and toss for about 30 seconds, or until fragrant. Remove from the heat.

4. Serve the stir-fry over the cooked rice.

Per serving: Calories: 312; Protein: 26g; Total fat: 6.5g; Saturated fat: 1g; Total carbohydrates: 37g; Fiber: 3.5g; Cholesterol: 159mg; Phosphorus: 320mg; Potassium: 581mg; Sodium: 604mg; Sugar: 10g

One-Pot Turkey Chili,
PAGE 114

POULTRY AND MEAT

One-Pot Turkey Chili ■

PREP TIME: 10 MINUTES • **COOK TIME:** 35 MINUTES • **SERVES** 4

Chili is the ultimate winter comfort food, and this one-pot meal is simple to prepare, easy to clean up, and is great for leftovers. For more spice, add a jalapeño pepper to this dish. Turkey is a cost-effective method for adding protein to the meal and the addition of kidney beans provides additional fiber. Top your chili with mozzarella (a low-phosphorus cheese) and a dollop of sour cream and fresh cilantro for a refreshing garnish.

1 tablespoon olive oil

1 medium white onion, minced

3 garlic cloves, minced

4 ounces turkey breast, cut into 1-inch pieces

2 cups chicken broth, no added salt

2 cups canned diced tomatoes, no added salt

1 cup canned white kidney beans, no added salt

1 tablespoon chili powder

1 tablespoon garlic powder

1 tablespoon ground cumin

1. In a large pot over medium heat, heat the olive oil. Add the onion and sauté until soft, about 10 minutes. Add the garlic and sauté for an additional minute.

2. In a medium-size skillet on medium heat, sauté the ground turkey until cooked, about 10 minutes until juices run translucent, then drain the excess fat. Add the turkey to the pot with onion.

3. Add the broth, tomatoes, beans, chili powder, garlic powder, and cumin to the pot and stir to combine. Bring to a boil, then reduce the heat to low and simmer for about 15 minutes, until the beans are heated through.

TIP: Leave out the ground turkey for a lower-protein and plant-based option.

Per serving: Calories: 182; Protein: 16g; Total fat: 4g; Saturated fat: 0.5g; Total carbohydrates: 20g; Fiber: 7g; Cholesterol: 14mg; Phosphorus: 96mg; Potassium: 577mg; Sodium: 98mg; Sugar: 4.5g

Sweet-and-Sour Meatballs ■

PREP TIME: 10 MINUTES • **COOK TIME:** 20 MINUTES • **SERVES** 4

These meatballs are great for dinner or a snack. Adding carrots, a low-potassium vegetable, into these meatballs helps keep them moist and adds extra fiber, color, and crunch. The homemade sweet-and-sour sauce for this recipe is quick and simple but packed with flavor.

5 ounces ground beef (93% lean)

1 tablespoon garlic powder

1 tablespoon onion powder

¼ cup old-fashioned rolled oats

½ cup grated carrot

1 large egg

2 cups Sweet-and-Sour Sauce (page 151)

ADAPT FOR CARDIOVASCULAR DISEASE:

Replace the ground beef with ground turkey for a lower-fat option.

1. Preheat the oven to 375°F. Line a baking sheet with parchment paper.

2. In a large bowl, combine the ground beef, garlic powder, onion powder, oats, carrot, and egg and mix well.

3. Shape the mixture into 1-inch balls. Place the meatballs on the prepared baking sheet, evenly spaced. Bake for 15 to 18 minutes, uncovered, until no longer pink.

4. In a large bowl, combine the meatballs and sauce, coating the meatballs completely. Serve immediately.

Per serving: Calories: 276; Protein: 12g; Total fat: 4g; Saturated fat: 1.5g; Total carbohydrates: 50g; Fiber: 2.5g; Cholesterol: 69mg; Phosphorus: 149mg; Potassium: 468mg; Sodium: 175mg; Sugar: 37g

Chicken Cacciatore ■

PREP TIME: 10 MINUTES • **COOK TIME:** 20 MINUTES • **SERVES** 4

Chicken thighs are a great source of lean protein, and in this meal they create a truly rustic and juicy dish that is full of classic Italian flavors like garlic, tomato, and parsley.

8 ounces dry spaghetti pasta

1 tablespoon olive oil

6 ounces skinless, boneless chicken thighs, halved

1 medium white onion, sliced

2 medium green bell peppers, sliced

1 (14.5-ounce) can diced tomatoes, no added salt

1 teaspoon garlic powder

1 teaspoon freshly ground black pepper

2 teaspoons dried parsley

ADAPT FOR CARDIOVASCULAR DISEASE:

Replace the chicken thighs with tofu for a heart-healthy option.

1. Cook the pasta according to the package directions. Drain and set aside.

2. Meanwhile, in a large pan over medium-high heat, heat the olive oil. Add the chicken, onion, and bell peppers and cook for 5 to 7 minutes, flipping halfway through cooking, until the chicken starts to turn opaque.

3. Add the tomatoes, garlic powder, pepper, and parsley to the pan, stirring to combine. Reduce the heat to low and simmer for about 10 minutes, until the chicken is cooked.

4. Remove the chicken from the heat and serve over the cooked pasta.

Per serving: Calories: 344; Protein: 17g; Total fat: 6.5g; Saturated fat: 1.5g; Total carbohydrates: 53g; Fiber: 4.5g; Cholesterol: 39mg; Phosphorus: 200mg; Potassium: 595mg; Sodium: 59mg; Sugar: 6.5g

Caribbean Seasoned Chicken ■

PREP TIME: 20 MINUTES • **COOK TIME:** 35 MINUTES • **SERVES** 4

Chicken thighs are a great source of iron and zinc, both of which are important for a healthy immune system. Soaking the chicken thighs in olive oil and lime juice keeps them juicy and provides vitamin C with a citrus hint. Serve this over rice.

6 ounces skinless, boneless chicken thighs, halved

2 tablespoons olive oil, divided

Juice of 2 limes

2½ tablespoons Caribbean Seasoning Mix (page 152)

1. Preheat the oven to 350°F. Line a baking sheet with aluminum foil.

2. On a plate, coat the chicken thighs in 1 tablespoon of olive oil and the lime juice.

3. Rub the Caribbean seasoning on the chicken and refrigerate for at least 15 minutes.

4. In a medium skillet, heat the remaining 1 tablespoon of olive oil over medium heat. Add the chicken and fry for 2 to 4 minutes per side, until browned.

5. Transfer the chicken to the prepared baking sheet. Bake for about 30 minutes, or until the juices run clear.

Per serving: Calories: 128; Protein: 8g; Total fat: 9.5g; Saturated fat: 1.5g; Total carbohydrates: 4g; Fiber: 1g; Cholesterol: 39mg; Phosphorus: 82mg; Potassium: 143mg; Sodium: 40mg; Sugar: 0.5g

Pork Tenderloin Stuffed with Apples and Onions ■

PREP TIME: 10 MINUTES • **COOK TIME:** 20 MINUTES • **SERVES** 4

Pork is a high-quality lean protein packed full of essential amino acids. This lean protein is considered a red meat because of its muscle structure, and it can be included in moderation in a kidney-friendly diet. When pork tenderloin is cooked with apples, it creates a flavorful and juicy experience. Inspired by fall flavors, this recipe is addictive.

1½ tablespoons olive oil, divided

2 teaspoons ground cinnamon

1 teaspoon freshly ground black pepper

1 teaspoon dried rosemary

1 pound pork tenderloin

1 medium white onion, cut into wedges

2 small apples, peeled, cored, and cut into wedges

1. Preheat the oven to 450°F. Lightly coat a roasting pan with 1 tablespoon of olive oil.

2. In a small bowl, mix the cinnamon, pepper, rosemary, and the remaining ½ tablespoon of olive oil. Place the spice mix on a plate and coat the pork with it.

3. Place the pork between the handles of two wooden spoons; the spoon handles will prevent slicing the pork all the way through. Slice the pork into 6 to 8 slices, leaving about ¼ inch at the bottom unsliced. Stuff the onion and apple wedges into each cut.

4. Place the tenderloin on the prepared roasting pan, cover it with aluminum foil, and roast for about 20 minutes, or until the pork is golden brown on the outside and the juices run clear. Remove from the oven and let rest for 5 minutes before serving.

Per serving: Calories: 229; Protein: 23g; Total fat: 8.5g; Saturated fat: 2g; Total carbohydrates: 17g; Fiber: 3.5g; Cholesterol: 61mg; Phosphorus: 244mg; Potassium: 507mg; Sodium: 50mg; Sugar: 11g

Chicken Stuffed Peppers ■

PREP TIME: 5 MINUTES • **COOK TIME:** 25 MINUTES • **SERVES** 4

Stuffed peppers are a great way to add extra fiber and color to a meal. This dinner recipe is one the entire family will love. Ground chicken is a low-fat protein that can be used in many recipes that traditionally call for ground beef. In this recipe, the chicken takes on the flavors of the spices and packs a flavor punch.

½ cup dry parboiled rice

4 large green bell peppers, tops cut off, seeded

2 tablespoons olive oil

1 medium white onion, chopped

5 ounces ground chicken

1 teaspoon chili powder

1 teaspoon paprika

1 teaspoon garlic powder

1 teaspoon onion powder

ADAPT FOR DIABETES:

Add extra fiber by including mushrooms or use bulgur instead of rice.

1. Cook the rice according to the package directions, usually about 25 minutes. Set aside.

2. Preheat the oven to 350°F. Place the bell peppers, cut-side up, in a small casserole dish.

3. In medium skillet, heat the olive oil over medium-high heat. Add the onion and chicken and cook for 6 to 8 minutes, until the chicken is cooked through. Drain the excess fat from the pan. Add the chili powder, paprika, garlic powder, and onion powder to the pan and mix to combine.

4. Add the rice to the chicken mixture and combine. Fill the bell peppers with equal amounts of the chicken mixture.

5. Bake, uncovered, until the peppers are tender, 20 to 25 minutes.

Per serving: Calories: 238; Protein: 10g; Total fat: 10g; Saturated fat: 2g; Total carbohydrates: 28g; Fiber: 3g; Cholesterol: 31mg; Phosphorus: 137mg; Potassium: 502mg; Sodium: 28mg; Sugar: 4g

Mediterranean Turkey Burgers ■

PREP TIME: 15 MINUTES • **COOK TIME:** 15 MINUTES • **SERVES** 4

Turkey burgers are a great lower-calorie alternative to beef burgers. Generally, turkey is lower in saturated fat than beef, and it includes healthy nutrients like niacin, selenium, B_6, and zinc. Onion, garlic, and rosemary pack a lot of flavor into these delicious and healthy turkey burgers. This recipe is great for entertaining or a weekend barbecue.

5 ounces ground turkey

1 teaspoon onion powder

1 teaspoon garlic powder

½ teaspoon freshly ground black pepper

1 tablespoon olive oil

1 tablespoon old-fashioned rolled oats

4 hamburger or brioche buns

Rosemary-Garlic Sauce (page 154)

1. In a medium bowl, combine the turkey, onion powder, garlic powder, pepper, olive oil, and oats. Mix well and shape into 4 patties.

2. Heat a medium skillet over medium-high heat. Grill the patties for about 5 minutes per side, or until fully cooked and the juices run clear.

3. Place a cooked patty on each bun and top with the sauce. Serve immediately.

TIP: Prepare the patties ahead of time and freeze, wrapped in plastic, for future meals.

Per serving: Calories: 245; Protein: 12g; Total fat: 10g; Saturated fat: 3g; Total carbohydrates: 25g; Fiber: 1.5g; Cholesterol: 34mg; Phosphorus: 118mg; Potassium: 155mg; Sodium: 246mg; Sugar: 4g

Buffalo Chicken ■

PREP TIME: 15 MINUTES • **COOK TIME:** 35 MINUTES • **SERVES** 4

This perfectly seasoned chicken is roasted in under one hour. Better than any chicken purchased from the deli section of the grocery store, this juicy treat is low in sodium and full of yummy spicy and tangy flavors.

¼ cup Buffalo Hot Sauce (page 155)

2 tablespoons olive oil

2 tablespoons dried rosemary

1 tablespoon freshly ground black pepper

1 tablespoon onion powder

1 tablespoon garlic powder

8 ounces skinless, boneless chicken breasts

1 celery stalk, halved

1 small white onion, halved

1 lemon, quartered

ADAPT FOR CKD STAGE 5:

Use 10-ounce chicken breasts for extra protein per serving.

1. Preheat the oven to 425°F.

2. In a small bowl, mix the Buffalo sauce, olive oil, rosemary, pepper, onion powder, and garlic powder.

3. In a roasting pan or casserole dish, cover the chicken with the sauce mixture and toss to coat.

4. Place the celery and onion around the chicken. Squeeze the lemon juice on the chicken, then place the lemon quarters in the roasting pan around the chicken.

5. Bake in the oven, uncovered, for about 35 minutes, or until the juices run clear. Serve immediately.

TIP: Use the leftover chicken for sandwiches or for topping salads and pasta dishes.

Per serving: Calories: 175; Protein: 14g; Total fat: 9.5g; Saturated fat: 2g; Total carbohydrates: 9g; Fiber: 2.5g; Cholesterol: 43mg; Phosphorus: 154mg; Potassium: 367mg; Sodium: 76mg; Sugar: 1.5g

Mushroom Chicken
with Rosemary and Thyme ■

PREP TIME: 15 MINUTES • **COOK TIME:** 35 MINUTES • **SERVES** 4

Mushrooms are a great source of fiber and antioxidants; however, they are often considered a high-potassium vegetable. Even so, mushrooms can be included in a kidney diet regardless of the stage or potassium restriction if serving size is considered.

5 ounces skinless, boneless chicken thighs, halved

½ teaspoon freshly ground black pepper

1 tablespoon olive oil

2 tablespoons unsalted butter, divided

1 cup sliced white button mushrooms

½ tablespoon dried parsley

½ teaspoon dried rosemary

½ teaspoon dried thyme

2 garlic cloves, minced

1. Coat the chicken pieces evenly with the pepper.

2. In a medium skillet over medium heat, heat the olive oil. Add the chicken and sear them until browned on each side and cooked through, about 8 minutes per side. The chicken is cooked when the juices run clear and no longer pink inside. Remove from the skillet and set aside.

3. In the same skillet, melt 1 tablespoon of butter and add the mushrooms. Season with the parsley, rosemary, and thyme and cook until the mushrooms are soft, about 10 minutes. Add the garlic and sauté for 1 minute. Add the remaining 1 tablespoon of butter.

4. Add the chicken and toss in the sauce to coat. Serve immediately.

Per serving: Calories: 130; Protein: 8g; Total fat: 11g; Saturated fat: 4.5g; Total carbohydrates: 2g; Fiber: 0.5g; Cholesterol: 44mg; Phosphorus: 21mg; Potassium: 75mg; Sodium: 34mg; Sugar: 0.5g

Pineapple-Glazed Chicken Thigh Stir-Fry ■

PREP TIME: 5 MINUTES • **COOK TIME:** 20 MINUTES • **SERVES** 4

This chicken stir-fry is tossed in a sweet and sticky sauce that has all the flavors of takeout with less salt and more fiber.

3 tablespoons olive oil, divided

2 medium green bell peppers, sliced

1 medium white onion, sliced

5 ounces skinless, boneless chicken thighs, cubed

2 tablespoons chopped fresh ginger

2 garlic cloves, minced

2 (8-ounce) cans juice-packed pineapple chunks

2 tablespoons reduced-sodium soy sauce

1 teaspoon red pepper flakes

2 cups cooked parboiled rice

ADAPT FOR CKD STAGE 5:

Try adding 7 ounces of firm tofu for extra protein.

1. In a medium skillet over medium heat, heat 1 tablespoon of olive oil. Add the bell peppers, and onion and sauté until the vegetables are cooked, about 5 minutes. Remove and set aside.

2. In the same pan, heat 1 tablespoon of olive oil. Add the chicken and cook fully, about 10 minutes. Remove the chicken and set aside with the vegetables.

3. In the same pan, heat the remaining 1 tablespoon of olive oil and sauté the ginger and garlic over medium-high heat, until fragrant. Add the pineapple, soy sauce, and red pepper flakes and stir to combine. Let the mixture bubble until slightly thickened.

4. Add the vegetables and cooked chicken to the pineapple sauce. Coat well until the chicken is covered with the sauce and warmed through.

5. Serve over the rice.

Per serving: Calories: 312; Protein: 12g; Total fat: 12g; Saturated fat: 2g; Total carbohydrates: 39g; Fiber: 3g; Cholesterol: 28mg; Phosphorus: 81mg; Potassium: 353mg; Sodium: 324mg; Sugar: 14g

Cottage Pie ■

PREP TIME: 15 MINUTES • **COOK TIME:** 40 MINUTES • **SERVES** 4

Traditional shepherd's pie is a British comfort food with ground lamb and vegetables. Cottage pie is equally as comforting but made with ground beef for extra health benefits like iron. The addition of the cauliflower to the mashed potatoes helps reduce the potassium and adds extra fiber, but the mixture still tastes like potatoes. Make ahead and freeze portions for a quick-and-easy leftover lunch. Use peas, carrots, and corn for the frozen vegetables.

8 ounces ground beef (93% lean)

2 cups frozen mixed vegetables

2 tablespoons dried rosemary

1 tablespoon dried thyme

½ cup beef broth, no added salt

½ medium cauliflower, chopped

1 small white potato, peeled and chopped

2 ounces plain cream cheese

ADAPT FOR CKD:

Replace the ground beef with canned lentils (no added salt) and vegetable broth (no added salt) for a plant-based option. For this option, add the lentils and broth to the skillet with the frozen vegetables, rosemary, and thyme and stir.

1. Preheat the oven to 350°F.

2. In a medium skillet over medium-high heat, brown the ground beef until cooked through, about 10 minutes. Drain the excess fat. Add the frozen vegetables, rosemary, thyme, and broth and stir to combine. Let simmer for 10 minutes.

3. Meanwhile, fill a large pot with water and bring to a boil. Add the cauliflower and potatoes and cook until tender, about 10 minutes. The potatoes and cauliflower should be tender when poked with a fork.

4. Drain the cauliflower and potato and return to the pot. Using a potato masher or blender, mash the cauliflower and potato together. Add the cream cheese and combine until smooth.

5. In a baking dish, place the meat mixture on the bottom. Top with the mashed cauliflower. Bake in the oven for about 20 minutes, or until the top is golden brown.

Per serving: Calories: 233; Protein: 17g; Total fat: 10g; Saturated fat: 4.5g; Total carbohydrates: 20g; Fiber: 5g; Cholesterol: 51mg; Phosphorus: 172mg; Potassium: 539mg; Sodium: 142mg; Sugar: 6g

Roasted Red Pepper Lasagna ■

PREP TIME: 15 MINUTES • **COOK TIME:** 1 HOUR 5 MINUTES • **SERVES** 4

Lasagna is a great food for meal prep because it can be made ahead of time and frozen for later use. This lasagna uses a homemade Red Pepper Sauce as a lower-potassium and lower-sodium option compared to traditional lasagna recipes.

Cooking spray

½ tablespoon olive oil

1 small white onion, minced

½ pound 92% lean, 8% fat ground beef

4 cups Roasted Red Pepper Sauce (page 149)

8 dry no-boil lasagna noodles

½ cup low-fat cottage cheese

¼ cup shredded part-skim mozzarella cheese

ADAPT FOR CARDIOVASCULAR DISEASE:

Swap out the ground beef for ground turkey or chicken for a lower-cholesterol option.

1. Preheat the oven to 375°F. Spray a loaf pan with cooking spray.

2. In a medium skillet, heat the olive oil. Add the onion and cook until soft, about 5 minutes. Add the ground beef and cook thoroughly, about 10 minutes. Drain the excess fat.

3. In the prepared loaf pan, add a layer of sauce, a layer of noodles, a layer of cottage cheese, and a layer of meat. Repeat until all the ingredients are used. Top with the mozzarella cheese and cover with aluminum foil.

4. Bake for 25 minutes. Remove the foil and bake for about 25 minutes, or until the cheese browns.

TIP: Add other vegetables, such as zucchini, spinach, or mushrooms, to the lasagna layers if potassium restriction is not a concern.

Per serving: Calories: 534; Protein: 27g; Total fat: 17g; Saturated fat: 4g; Total carbohydrates: 65g; Fiber: 7g; Cholesterol: 41mg; Phosphorus: 269mg; Potassium: 723mg; Sodium: 589mg; Sugar: 14g

Taco-Flavored Beef and Rice Soup ■

PREP TIME: 5 MINUTES • **COOK TIME:** 50 MINUTES • **SERVES** 4

A low-sodium twist on the traditional beef soup, this meal includes hints of chili and cumin, and it will send the taste buds singing. This rich soup can be prepared ahead of time and frozen for a quick weeknight meal.

2 tablespoons olive oil

½ pound lean stew beef, cut into 1-inch cubes

1 medium white onion, diced

2 medium celery stalks, diced

2 garlic cloves, minced

2 medium carrots, diced

2 tablespoons Taco Seasoning (page 153)

1 teaspoon freshly ground black pepper

½ cup dry parboiled rice

4 cups beef broth, no added salt

3 cups water

ADAPT FOR STAGES 1 TO 4:

For a lower-protein option, decrease the beef to ¼ pound.

1. In a large pot over medium-high heat, heat the olive oil. Add the beef and sear for 2 minutes per side. Remove and set aside.

2. In the same pot, add the onion, celery, garlic, carrots, and seasoning. Cook for about 5 minutes, or until the vegetables are tender.

3. Add the pepper, rice, broth, water, and beef to the pot. Cover and cook for 30 to 40 minutes, until the beef and rice are tender. Serve immediately.

TIP: The homemade taco seasoning can be replaced with a packaged low-sodium taco seasoning.

Per serving: Calories: 342; Protein: 22g; Total fat: 15g; Saturated fat: 4g; Total carbohydrates: 28g; Fiber: 2.5g; Cholesterol: 60mg; Phosphorus: 198mg; Potassium: 407mg; Sodium: 355mg; Sugar: 3g

Taco-Flavored Meat Casserole ■

PREP TIME: 15 MINUTES • **COOK TIME:** 40 MINUTES • **SERVES** 4

This Mexican-inspired casserole is loaded with flavors, easy to assemble, and packed with fiber from the beans. Top this dish with crispy and fresh vegetables like lettuce, tomato, and peppers for a balanced meal.

½ pound ground beef (93% lean)

1 small white onion, chopped

2 tablespoons Taco Seasoning (page 153)

1½ cups black beans, no added salt

½ cup water

1 cup shredded cheddar cheese

1 cup crumbled low-sodium tortilla chips

2 scallions, chopped (white and green parts)

2 cups chopped lettuce

¼ cup diced tomatoes

½ cup diced green bell peppers

1 cup Enchilada Sauce (page 150)

ADAPT FOR HYPERTENSION:

Reduce the sodium by using the Homemade Flour Tortillas (page 147) instead of the low-sodium tortilla chips.

1. Preheat the oven to 350°F.

2. In a large pan over medium heat, cook the ground beef and onion until the beef is cooked through, about 10 minutes. Drain the excess fat.

3. Add the seasoning, black beans, and water to the pan. Bring to a simmer and cook until the liquid has been reduced by half, about 15 minutes.

4. Spread the bean and meat mixture on the bottom of a casserole dish and top with the cheese. Bake, uncovered, for about 15 minutes, or until the cheese is melted.

5. Top with the tortilla chips, scallions, lettuce, tomatoes, and bell peppers and drizzle the sauce on the top before serving.

TIP: When time is an issue, use store-bought hot sauce, packaged taco seasoning, and tortillas.

Per serving: Calories: 361; Protein: 26g; Total fat: 16g; Saturated fat: 7g; Total carbohydrates: 28g; Fiber: 7.5g; Cholesterol: 64mg; Phosphorus: 357mg; Potassium: 657mg; Sodium: 294mg; Sugar: 3g

Lemon-Thyme Pork Tenderloin ■

PREP TIME: 10 MINUTES • **COOK TIME:** 20 MINUTES • **SERVES** 4

Pork tenderloin is a cost-effective protein, and with very little work, it can become a juicy and delicious meal. The lemon juice, garlic, and thyme create a simple and flavorful marinade.

4 tablespoons lemon juice

1 tablespoon olive oil

2 teaspoons dried thyme

2 teaspoons garlic powder

1 teaspoon freshly ground black pepper

8 ounces pork tenderloin

ADAPT FOR CARDIOVASCULAR DISEASE:

Pork tenderloin is one of the leanest cuts of pork, but still be sure to trim off the visible fat.

1. Preheat the oven to 425°F. Line a baking sheet with aluminum foil.

2. In a small bowl, mix the lemon juice, olive oil, thyme, garlic powder, and pepper.

3. Coat the pork tenderloin with the mixture and place on the prepared baking sheet. Roast for 15 to 20 minutes, until golden brown on the outside and the juices run clear.

Per serving: Calories: 102; Protein: 11g; Total fat: 5g; Saturated fat: 1g; Total carbohydrates: 3g; Fiber: 0.5g; Cholesterol: 31mg; Phosphorus: 121mg; Potassium: 222mg; Sodium: 25mg; Sugar: 0.5g

Beef Bourguignon ◼

PREP TIME: 10 MINUTES • **COOK TIME:** 25 MINUTES • **SERVES** 4

Beef bourguignon is a classic French beef stew made of meat that is slowly simmered in red wine, onions, mushrooms, and crisp bacon. With this version, the wine and bacon are eliminated, but the hearty tomato paste, red wine vinegar, onion, and garlic flavors will still make any mouth water. This dish is best served with Garlic Double-Boiled Mashed Potatoes (page 66) or roasted carrots for a low-potassium side dish.

1 pound boneless beef sirloin steak, cut into 1-inch cubes

2 teaspoons freshly ground black pepper, divided

2 tablespoons olive oil, divided

½ cup canned diced tomatoes, no added salt

1 tablespoon tomato paste, no added salt

1 small white onion, sliced

1 garlic clove, minced

1 cup beef broth, no added salt

½ cup red wine vinegar

1 teaspoon chili powder

1. Season the beef cubes with 1 teaspoon of pepper. In a medium skillet over medium heat, heat 1 tablespoon of olive oil. Add the beef and cook for 2 to 3 minutes, until the outside is browned but still rare inside. Remove and set aside.

2. Heat the remaining 1 tablespoon of olive oil in the same skillet. Add the tomatoes, tomato paste, onion, garlic, broth, red wine vinegar, chili powder, and the remaining 1 teaspoon of pepper. Bring to a boil. Reduce the heat to low and simmer for 5 minutes.

3. Add the beef back to skillet, and cook for about 10 more minutes, or until the beef is medium rare. Add more time for desired doneness. Serve immediately.

Per serving: Calories: 237; Protein: 27g; Total fat: 12g; Saturated fat: 2.5g; Total carbohydrates: 5g; Fiber: 1g; Cholesterol: 80mg; Phosphorus: 265mg; Potassium: 614mg; Sodium: 117mg; Sugar: 2g

DESSERTS

Apple Crisp ■

PREP TIME: 10 MINUTES • **COOK TIME:** 50 MINUTES • **SERVES** 6

Apples are a great high-fiber and low-potassium fruit. Cinnamon, honey, and apples come together to make this light and refreshing apple crisp, a true fall dessert. Use tart apples such as Granny Smith, Honeycrisp, or Golden Delicious.

Cooking spray

6 apples, skin on, cored, and cubed

2 tablespoons honey, plus ½ cup

2 tablespoons ground cinnamon, divided

2 teaspoons lemon juice

¾ cup old-fashioned rolled oats

¾ cup all-purpose flour

½ cup unsalted butter, cold, diced

ADAPT FOR DIABETES:

Reduce the honey in the crumble topping to ¼ cup.

1. Preheat the oven to 350°F. Spray an 8-by-8-inch baking dish with cooking spray.

2. In a medium bowl, combine the apples, 2 tablespoons of honey, 1 tablespoon of cinnamon, and the lemon juice and mix well. Pour the mixture into the prepared baking dish.

3. In a another medium bowl, combine the ½ cup of honey, the oats, flour, the remaining 1 tablespoon of cinnamon, and the butter. Using a pastry cutter or two butter knives, cut the butter into the topping mixture, until it looks like pea-size crumbs.

4. Spread the topping over the apples in the baking dish. Bake for 40 to 50 minutes, until bubbling and golden brown.

Per serving: Calories: 424; Protein: 4g; Total fat: 19g; Saturated fat: 10g; Total carbohydrates: 67g; Fiber: 6g; Cholesterol: 41mg; Phosphorus: 80mg; Potassium: 269mg; Sodium: 5mg; Sugar: 41g

Shortbread Cookies ■

PREP TIME: 10 MINUTES • **COOK TIME:** 20 MINUTES • **MAKES** 24 COOKIES

These easy-to-make cookies melt in the mouth and are a great staple recipe for the holidays. They come together with only four ingredients and can be made quickly when unexpected guests turn up. Shortbread cookies are a great kidney-friendly option as they are low in phosphorus.

1 cup unsalted butter, room temperature

⅓ cup honey

2 teaspoons vanilla extract

2½ cups all-purpose flour

ADAPT FOR CARDIOVASCULAR DISEASE:

Use plant-sterol-enriched margarine instead of the unsalted butter.

1. Preheat the oven to 350°F.

2. In a medium bowl, using a hand mixer, cream the butter, honey, and vanilla. Mix until creamy.

3. Add the flour, ½ cup at a time, into the butter mixture and continue mixing, until the dough comes together.

4. Using 1 teaspoon of the batter, form the dough into balls and place on a nonstick baking sheet.

5. When all the dough is formed, you should have 24 balls. Bake for 15 to 20 minutes, until lightly golden brown.

Per serving (2 cookies): Calories: 260; Protein: 3g; Total fat: 16g; Saturated fat: 9.5g; Total carbohydrates: 28g; Fiber: 0,5g; Cholesterol: 41mg; Phosphorus: 33mg; Potassium: 38mg; Sodium: 3mg; Sugar: 7g

Oatmeal Cookies ■

PREP TIME: 10 MINUTES • **COOK TIME:** 15 MINUTES • **MAKES** 32 COOKIES

A classic comfort food, no cookie can compete. This cookie is perfectly spiced with cinnamon to bring back childhood memories. The addition of almonds, walnuts, or dried cranberries creates different variations on this recipe.

1½ cups all-purpose flour

2 teaspoons ground cinnamon

¾ teaspoon Baking Powder Substitute (page 146)

¼ teaspoon salt

1 cup unsalted butter, room temperature

1 cup honey

2 large eggs

2 teaspoons vanilla extract

3 cups old-fashioned rolled oats

1. Preheat the oven to 350°F. Line three full-size baking sheets with parchment paper.

2. In a medium bowl, whisk together the flour, cinnamon, Baking Powder Substitute, and salt.

3. In a second medium bowl, cream together the butter and honey with a hand mixer. Mix in 1 egg. Once blended, mix in the remaining egg and the vanilla.

4. Add the flour mixture to the egg mixture and mix just until combined. Add the oats and mix to combine.

5. Scoop out the dough, shape it into 1½-inch balls, and place the balls on the prepared baking sheets, fitting 12 per sheet and spacing 2 inches apart.

6. Bake in the oven until the edges are golden brown, about 12 to 15 minutes.

7. Let cool on the baking sheets for a few minutes, then transfer to a wire rack to cool completely.

Per serving (2 cookies): Calories: 276; Protein: 4g; Total fat: 13g; Saturated fat: 7.5g; Total carbohydrates: 36g; Fiber: 2g; Cholesterol: 54mg; Phosphorus: 86mg; Potassium: 109mg; Sodium: 67mg; Sugar: 16g

Rice Pudding ■

PREP TIME: 5 MINUTES • **COOK TIME:** 40 MINUTES • **SERVES** 4

This old-fashioned rice pudding is creamy, decadent, and sweet. Use of the almond milk is a kidney-friendly twist. With only a few ingredients needed, this is a snap to make on busy days. It is typically topped with dried raisins, but feel free to try other delicious alternatives, such as fresh berries, bananas, or dried cranberries.

½ cup dry parboiled rice

4 cups unsweetened plain almond milk

1 tablespoon honey

2 teaspoons vanilla extract

2 teaspoons ground cinnamon

1. In a medium heavy saucepan over medium heat, bring the rice, almond milk, honey, and vanilla to a simmer, stirring often.

2. Reduce the heat to low, cover, and simmer, stirring occasionally, for 25 minutes, or until the pudding is slightly thickened; Divide among 4 bowls and let it cool in the refrigerator; it will thicken more as it cools.

3. Before eating, sprinkle each serving with the cinnamon.

TIP: For a chocolate rice pudding, add 2 teaspoons of cocoa powder. Try adding more fiber by adding fresh fruits, like blueberries or raspberries, when serving.

Per serving: Calories: 89; Protein: 2g; Total fat: 3g; Saturated fat: 0g; Total carbohydrates: 12g; Fiber: 1g; Cholesterol: 0mg; Phosphorus: 38mg; Potassium: 198mg; Sodium: 187mg; Sugar: 4.5g

Blondies ◾

PREP TIME: 10 MINUTES • **COOK TIME:** 30 MINUTES • **MAKES** 12 BARS

Cranberries are a low-potassium fruit that are also a great source of anti-oxidants and vitamin C and help support immune function. These white chocolate blondies are soft, buttery, and filled with tart cranberries to balance the flavors in this delicious treat.

Cooking spray

¾ cup unsalted butter, melted

1 cup honey

1 large egg

1 teaspoon vanilla extract

1½ cups all-purpose flour

1 cup fresh cranberries

½ cup white chocolate chips

ADAPT FOR DIABETES:

Substitute the honey for an artificial sweetener like Splenda in a one-to-one ratio.

1. Preheat the oven to 325°F. Coat an 8-by-8-inch baking pan with cooking spray.

2. In a large bowl, combine the butter and honey.

3. Add the egg and vanilla and mix until combined.

4. Stir in the flour. Then fold in the cranberries and white chocolate chips.

5. Pour the batter into the prepared pan. Place in the oven and bake for about 30 minutes, or until golden brown around the edges. Leave in the pan to cool completely.

6. When cool, cut into 12 squares and serve.

Per serving (1 bar): Calories: 300; Protein: 3g; Total fat: 15g; Saturated fat: 9g; Total carbohydrates: 40g; Fiber: 0.5g; Cholesterol: 48mg; Phosphorus: 43mg; Potassium: 67mg; Sodium: 15mg; Sugar: 26g

Key Lime Mini Desserts ■

PREP TIME: 15 MINUTES, PLUS 1 HOUR TO CHILL •
COOK TIME: 10 MINUTES • **SERVES** 8

This easy-to-make dessert is tart and sweet. The crunchy graham cracker crust is filled with a creamy chia seed pudding balanced with limes. The chia seeds add fiber, which makes these small dessert portions very filling.

5 tablespoons unsalted butter, melted

1¼ cups graham cracker crumbs

8 tablespoons chia seeds

2 cups unsweetened plain almond milk

2 tablespoons lime juice

½ teaspoon vanilla extract

1. Preheat the oven to 350°F.

2. Mix the butter and graham crackers in a small bowl. Arrange 8 small oven-safe ramekins on a baking sheet and press the graham crust into the cups, filling each halfway. Bake for 10 minutes. Remove from the oven and let cool.

3. While the crust is baking, in a medium bowl combine the chia seeds, almond milk, lime juice, and vanilla.

4. Divide the pudding among the cooled ramekins, and place in the refrigerator for 30 to 60 minutes to thicken. Leave the chia seed pudding for as long as possible to make a thicker pudding.

TIP: Swap out the lime for lemon for a citrus alternative.

Per serving: Calories: 193; Protein: 3g; Total fat: 13g; Saturated fat: 5g; Total carbohydrates: 17g; Fiber: 4g; Cholesterol: 19mg; Phosphorus: 128mg; Potassium: 120mg; Sodium: 121mg; Sugar: 4g

Big Soft Ginger Cookies ■

PREP TIME: 5 MINUTES • **COOK TIME:** 10 MINUTES • **MAKES** 12 COOKIES

Ginger is known for improving digestion, reducing inflammation, and supporting cardiovascular health. These cookies are perfectly spiced and supersoft.

2¼ cups all-purpose flour

2 teaspoons
  ground ginger

1 teaspoon baking soda

1 teaspoon ground
  cinnamon

¾ cup unsalted butter,
  room temperature

1 cup honey

¼ cup water

1 large egg

1. Preheat the oven to 350°F.

2. In a medium bowl, mix the flour, ginger, baking soda, and cinnamon and set aside.

3. In a separate large bowl, beat the butter with an electric mixer on medium speed for 30 seconds. Add the honey and combine. Add the water and egg and combine.

4. Stir the dry ingredients into the egg mixture until it forms a dough.

5. Shape the dough into ½-inch balls, using about 2 tablespoons of dough for each ball.

6. Place the balls about 2½ inches apart on an ungreased baking sheet.

7. Bake for about 10 minutes, or until the cookies are light brown and puffed. Let the cookies stand on the baking sheet for about 2 minutes before transferring them to a wire rack to cool completely.

TIP: These cookies are the perfect texture to make whoopie pies. Simply use two cookies and make a sandwich filled with whipped topping.

Per serving (1 cookie): Calories: 280; Protein: 3g; Total fat: 12g; Saturated fat: 7.5g; Total carbohydrates: 41g; Fiber: 1g; Cholesterol: 46mg; Phosphorus: 39mg; Potassium: 53mg; Sodium: 114mg; Sugar: 21g

Cinnamon Rolls ■

PREP TIME: 10 MINUTES • **COOK TIME:** 25 MINUTES
MAKES 9 CINNAMON ROLLS

These are the quickest and easiest cinnamon rolls to make. If gooey cinnamon rolls that melt in the mouth are desired, this recipe is perfect. Because the traditional yeast found in cinnamon rolls is omitted, these rolls are now a kidney-friendly option that is also low in potassium. Best if enjoyed warm.

Cooking spray

For the dough:

2 cups all-purpose flour, plus more for dusting

¾ teaspoon salt

5 tablespoons unsalted butter, cold

¾ cup unsweetened plain almond milk

1 large egg

For the filling:

3 tablespoons ground cinnamon

¼ cup honey

¼ cup unsalted butter, room temperature

For the frosting:

½ cup plain cream cheese, room temperature

3 tablespoons unsalted butter, room temperature

1 teaspoon vanilla extract

To make the dough:

1. Preheat the oven to 350°F. Grease a 9-by-9-inch baking dish with cooking spray.

2. In a large bowl, combine the flour, salt, and butter using a pastry cutter or two knives to cut the butter into the flour.

3. Add the almond milk and egg. Mix well until the dough forms a ball.

4. Dump the dough onto a well-floured surface and roll until it forms a cohesive ball. Continue to dust the surface while working if needed. Use a rolling pin to flatten the ball into a 9-by-11-inch rectangle.

To make the filling:

5. In a small bowl, mix the cinnamon, honey, and butter. Spread the mixture over the dough, leaving a ¼-inch margin at the far side of the dough.

6. Tightly roll the dough into a tube and cut it into 9 (1-inch) sections.

continued ▶

CINNAMON ROLLS *continued*

ADAPT FOR DIABETES:

For a low-sugar alternative, use an artificial sweetener like Splenda instead of honey. Splenda can be substituted one-to-one for honey in this recipe.

7. Place the cinnamon rolls, with the filling showing on top, in the prepared baking dish. Bake for 20 to 25 minutes, or until just slightly golden brown on the edges. Remove from the oven and let cool for 5 minutes.

To make the frosting:

8. In a medium bowl, using a hand mixer, combine the cream cheese, butter, and vanilla until smooth and fluffy. Spread the cream cheese mixture over the cinnamon rolls. Enjoy.

Per serving (1 roll): Calories: 342; Protein: 5g; Total fat: 21g; Saturated fat: 12g; Total carbohydrates: 34g; Fiber: 2g; Cholesterol: 74mg; Phosphorus: 67mg; Potassium: 94mg; Sodium: 261mg; Sugar: 8g

Lemon Loaf ■

PREP TIME: 5 MINUTES • **COOK TIME:** 50 MINUTES • **SERVES** 12

Lemons are a low-potassium citrus fruit packed with vitamin C. This lemon loaf is rich with lemon flavor. It tastes just like something from a coffee shop but has all the kidney-friendly modifications.

Cooking spray

1 cup all-purpose flour

½ teaspoon baking soda

2 tablespoons lemon zest

4 large eggs

½ cup honey

½ cup unsweetened applesauce

½ cup olive oil

½ cup lemon juice, plus ½ tablespoon

1 teaspoon vanilla extract

½ cup powdered sugar

½ tablespoon unsweetened almond milk

ADAPT FOR CARDIOVASCULAR DISEASE:

Substitute ½ cup egg whites for 2 eggs.

1. Preheat the oven to 350°F. Coat a loaf pan with cooking spray.

2. In a medium bowl, whisk together the flour, baking soda, and lemon zest.

3. In a separate medium bowl, whisk together the eggs, honey, applesauce, olive oil, ½ cup of lemon juice and the vanilla.

4. Add the dry ingredients to the egg mixture and fold them together with a spoon.

5. Pour the batter into the prepared loaf pan and bake for about 50 minutes, or until the loaf is golden brown and a toothpick inserted in the center comes out clean. Remove from the oven and let cool.

6. In a small bowl, whisk together the powdered sugar, ½ tablespoon of lemon juice, and the almond milk until smooth.

7. Once the loaf is cool, spread the icing evenly over the top with a butter knife.

8. Cut into 12 slices.

Per serving (1 slice): Calories: 218; Protein: 3g; Total fat: 12g; Saturated fat: 2g; Total carbohydrates: 26g; Fiber: 0.5g; Cholesterol: 62mg; Phosphorus: 46mg; Potassium: 62mg; Sodium: 77mg; Sugar: 17g

Vanilla-Lemon Cookies ▪

PREP TIME: 10 MINUTES • **COOK TIME:** 15 MINUTES • **MAKES** 24 COOKIES

Sugar cookies are often made with sugar and baking powder, but for this kidney-friendly twist, the flavor comes from the honey and lemon instead. This twist on a sugar cookie packs a crispy lemon crunch and will put a smile on every face. These cookies are bursting with lemon flavor but lack the tartness.

1 cup unsalted butter, room temperature

1½ cups honey

2 large eggs

1 teaspoon vanilla extract

3 tablespoons lemon juice

3 cups all-purpose flour

¾ teaspoon Baking Powder Substitute (page 146)

½ teaspoon salt

ADAPT FOR DIABETES:

To reduce the sugar content, substitute 2 cups Splenda for the honey.

1. Preheat the oven to 325°F.

2. In a medium bowl, using a hand mixer, cream together the butter and honey until light and fluffy. Add the eggs, vanilla, and lemon juice and mix to combine.

3. Add the flour, Baking Powder Substitute, and salt. Mix to combine well.

4. Roll the dough into 1-inch balls and place them on a baking sheet. Bake in the oven for 9 to 12 minutes, until golden brown on the bottom.

Per serving (2 cookies): Calories: 391; Protein: 5g; Total fat: 16g; Saturated fat: 10g; Total carbohydrates: 58g; Fiber: 1g; Cholesterol: 72mg; Phosphorus: 57mg; Potassium: 96mg; Sodium: 139mg; Sugar: 32g

Homemade Flour Tortillas, PAGE 147

CHAPTER 9

HOMEMADE STAPLES

Baking Powder Substitute ■ ■ ■

PREP TIME: 5 MINUTES • **MAKES** 1 TABLESPOON

Baking powder is a leavening agent to help baked products rise. With CKD it can be a source of sodium and phosphorus. Too much phosphorus can be dangerous for individuals with CKD, because it can cause bones and teeth to become weak. One strategy to minimize phosphorus when baking is to use a baking powder substitute. This recipe substitution is for 1 tablespoon of baking powder, and it can be used to make other recipes kidney-friendly by swapping self-rising flour and using this substitute with all-purpose flour, so compare to what your recipe requires.

2 teaspoons cream
  of tartar

1 teaspoon baking soda

In a small bowl, combine the cream of tartar and baking soda.

TIP: Make a large batch and store in the pantry for future use.

Per serving (1 teaspoon): Calories: 5; Protein: 0g; Total fat: 0g; Saturated fat: 0g; Total carbohydrates: 1g; Fiber: 0g; Cholesterol: 0mg; Phosphorus: 0mg; Potassium: 330mg; Sodium: 420mg; Sugar: 0g

Homemade Flour Tortillas ▪ ▪ ▪

PREP TIME: 5 MINUTES • **COOK TIME:** 15 MINUTES • **MAKES** 8 TORTILLAS

Homemade tortillas are much lower in sodium and phosphorus than store-bought tortillas because the amount of salt is less and the baking powder can be omitted. These flour tortillas are soft and tender and have a light flavor. Prepare them ahead of time and store them in an airtight container separated with parchment paper.

2 cups all-purpose flour, plus more as needed

½ teaspoon salt

¾ cup hot water

2 tablespoons olive oil

ADAPT FOR DIABETES:

Use a mixture of 1 cup whole-grain flour and 1 cup all-purpose flour for a higher-fiber tortilla.

1. In a medium bowl, mix the flour and salt. Carefully add the hot water and olive oil and let it cool until safe to mix. When cool, mix the dough by hand for about 2 minutes.

2. Once the dough is mixed, knead on the counter and form into a ball. Add extra flour to the counter to prevent sticking if needed. Divide the dough into 8 balls and roll out each ball into 8-inch thin tortillas.

3. Heat a medium skillet over medium-high heat. Cook each tortilla 1 to 2 minutes on each side, until golden brown and soft. Use a large spatula to flip the tortillas.

Per serving (1 tortilla): Calories: 144; Protein: 3g; Total fat: 3.5g; Saturated fat: 0.5g; Total carbohydrates: 24g; Fiber: 1g; Cholesterol: 0mg; Phosphorus: 34mg; Potassium: 33mg; Sodium: 146mg; Sugar: 0g

Stir-Fry Sauce ■ ■ ■

PREP TIME: 5 MINUTES • **COOK TIME:** 10 MINUTES • **MAKES** ABOUT 1¼ CUPS

This stir-fry sauce is flavorful and easy to prepare, and it will become a staple in the refrigerator. It is sodium reduced but still packed with flavor from the garlic, ginger, and beef broth. This recipe can be made ahead and stored in the refrigerator in an airtight container for one week.

¼ cup reduced-sodium soy sauce

¾ cup beef broth, no added salt

2 tablespoons honey

2 tablespoons white vinegar

2 teaspoons garlic powder

1 teaspoon ground ginger

1. In a medium pot over medium heat, combine the soy sauce, broth, honey, vinegar, garlic powder, and ginger and stir together.

2. Let simmer for 5 to 8 minutes, until thickened.

TIP: Add sesame oil at the end of cooking for an extra umami flavor.

Per serving (¼ cup): Calories: 42; Protein: 2g; Total fat: 0g; Saturated fat: 0g; Total carbohydrates: 9g; Fiber: 0g; Cholesterol: 0mg; Phosphorus: 28mg; Potassium: 69mg; Sodium: 473mg; Sugar: 6.5g

Roasted Red Pepper Sauce ■ ■ ■

PREP TIME: 5 MINUTES • **MAKES** ABOUT 2 CUPS

A low-potassium sauce option, with all the flavor of tomato sauce. This marinara alternative is great with pasta or chicken or on pizza.

3 jarred roasted
  red peppers

2 garlic cloves, minced

1 cup no-salt-added
  tomato sauce

1 tablespoon olive oil

2 teaspoons
  dried oregano

1 teaspoon freshly
  ground black pepper

ADAPT FOR CKD:

Try roasting the red peppers by placing them on a baking sheet in the oven at 450°F for 15 to 20 minutes, until the skins are blackened.

1. In a blender, puree the red peppers, garlic, tomato sauce, olive oil, oregano, and pepper together.

2. Use immediately or place in the refrigerator in an airtight container for later use.

TIP: The sauce can be frozen in a freezer-safe airtight container for up to 3 months.

Per serving (½ cup): Calories: 90; Protein: 1g; Total fat: 3.5g; Saturated fat: 0.5g; Total carbohydrates: 12g; Fiber: 2.5g; Cholesterol: 0mg; Phosphorus: 4mg; Potassium: 208mg; Sodium: 194mg; Sugar: 6g

Enchilada Sauce ■ ■ ■

PREP TIME: 5 MINUTES • **COOK TIME:** 10 MINUTES • **MAKES** 2½ CUPS

Ready in under 20 minutes, this sauce makes store-bought enchilada sauce a thing of the past. Packed with flavor, featuring a slight spicy punch, and low in sodium, this sauce will be a favorite for any dish that needs a little spicy kick.

3 tablespoons all-purpose flour

1 tablespoon chili powder

1 teaspoon ground cumin

1 teaspoon garlic powder

½ teaspoon paprika

½ teaspoon ground cinnamon

2 tablespoons low-sodium tomato paste

2 cups vegetable broth, no added salt

1 teaspoon white vinegar

1. In a medium pot over medium heat, combine the flour, chili powder, cumin, garlic powder, paprika, and cinnamon. Stir constantly until fragrant, about 1 minute.

2. Add the tomato paste and then slowly stir in the broth. Continue stirring for about 5 minutes, or until the sauce is thickened.

3. Remove from the heat and stir in the vinegar.

TIP: The sauce can be stored in an airtight container in the refrigerator for up to 2 days.

Per serving (½ cup): Calories: 36; Protein: 1g; Total fat: 0g; Saturated fat: 0g; Total carbohydrates: 7g; Fiber: 1g; Cholesterol: 0mg; Phosphorus: 14mg; Potassium: 84mg; Sodium: 73mg; Sugar: 1.5g

Sweet-and-Sour Sauce ■ ■ ■

PREP TIME: 5 MINUTES • **COOK TIME:** 10 MINUTES • **MAKES** 2½ CUPS

This recipe is essential for any household. The sweet, sour, and tangy flavors come together to make a rich and tasty sauce. Use this sauce on meatballs or as a dip with chicken fingers.

½ cup honey

½ cup rice vinegar

2 tablespoons low-sodium tomato paste

1 tablespoon reduced-sodium soy sauce

2 (8-ounce) cans juice-packed pineapple chunks

1 medium green bell pepper, chopped

1. In a medium pot over medium-high heat, combine the honey, vinegar, tomato paste, soy sauce, and pineapple. Bring to a boil.

2. Stir in the bell pepper. Let simmer for about 10 minutes, or until the pepper is tender and the sauce is thick.

TIP: Canned pineapple is convenient for this recipe, but if fresh pineapple is available, that can be used instead.

TIP: The sauce can be stored in an airtight container in the refrigerator for up to 2 days.

Per serving (¼ cup): Calories: 83; Protein: 1g; Total fat: 0g; Saturated fat: 0g; Total carbohydrates: 21g; Fiber: 0.5g; Cholesterol: 0mg; Phosphorus: 9mg; Potassium: 112mg; Sodium: 61mg; Sugar: 18g

Caribbean Seasoning Mix ■ ■ ■

PREP TIME: 5 MINUTES • **MAKES** ¼ CUP

Spicy flavors from the Caribbean add punch and sizzle to this staple item. This seasoning can be used in many ways. Try flavoring proteins, adding it to rice, or spicing up roasted vegetables.

1 tablespoon
onion powder

1 tablespoon
garlic powder

2 teaspoons chili powder

2 teaspoons paprika

1 teaspoon freshly ground
black pepper

½ teaspoon ground cumin

½ teaspoon ground
cinnamon

1. In a small bowl, combine the onion powder, garlic powder, chili powder, paprika, pepper, cumin, and cinnamon.

2. Use immediately or store in the pantry in an air-tight container for up to 6 months.

Per serving (1 tablespoon): Calories: 21; Protein: 1g; Total fat: 0g; Saturated fat: 0g; Total carbohydrates: 5g; Fiber: 1.5g; Cholesterol: 0mg; Phosphorus: 20mg; Potassium: 81mg; Sodium: 14mg; Sugar: 0.5g

Taco Seasoning ■ ■ ■

PREP TIME: 5 MINUTES • **MAKES** ¼ CUP

This seasoning can be used as a dry rub, mixed with sour cream as a dip, or used to flavor tacos or fajitas. By making this seasoning at home and not buying it in the store, the amount of sodium can be reduced.

2 tablespoons chili powder

4 teaspoons ground cumin

1 teaspoon onion powder

1 teaspoon garlic powder

1 teaspoon dried parsley

1 teaspoon paprika

1. In a bowl, combine the chili powder, cumin, onion powder, garlic powder, parsley, and paprika.

2. Use immediately or store in the pantry in an airtight container for up to 6 months.

TIP: Add cayenne powder for extra spice.

Per serving (1 tablespoon): Calories: 16; Protein: 1g; Total fat: 0.5g; Saturated fat: 0g; Total carbohydrates: 2g; Fiber: 1g; Cholesterol: 0mg; Phosphorus: 7mg; Potassium: 32mg; Sodium: 36mg; Sugar: 0g

Rosemary-Garlic Sauce ■ ■ ■

PREP TIME: 5 MINUTES • **MAKES** ¼ CUP

This sour cream dip is great served with turkey burgers or fish or used for dipping vegetables or crackers. Rosemary is an herbaceous shrub that originated in the Mediterranean that can be grown easily on the kitchen counter or in the backyard. It can almost always be found in the grocery store as well, so it's enjoyable all year long.

¼ cup sour cream

1 garlic clove, minced

2 teaspoons lemon juice

1 teaspoon dried rosemary

½ teaspoon freshly ground black pepper

ADAPT FOR CARDIOVASCULAR DISEASE:

Use plain low-fat yogurt instead of sour cream.

1. In a small bowl, mix the sour cream, garlic, lemon juice, rosemary, and pepper.

2. Use immediately or store in the refrigerator in an airtight container for up to 1 week.

Per serving (1 tablespoon): Calories: 33; Protein: 1g; Total fat: 2.5g; Saturated fat: 1.5g; Total carbohydrates: 2g; Fiber: 0g; Cholesterol: 10mg; Phosphorus: 2mg; Potassium: 12mg; Sodium: 8mg; Sugar: 0.5g

Buffalo Hot Sauce ■■■

PREP TIME: 5 MINUTES • **COOK TIME:** 40 MINUTES • **MAKES** 2 CUPS

This low-sodium hot sauce is easy to prepare and packed with heat. Use with the Spicy Buffalo Cauliflower Bites (page 68) or as a dip for chicken or fish. Prepare ahead of time to let it marinate as this sauce takes on flavors the longer it sits.

18 fresh cayenne peppers, ends removed and finely chopped

1½ cups white vinegar

4 teaspoons garlic powder

½ teaspoon salt

½ teaspoon freshly ground black pepper

2 tablespoons unsalted butter

1. In a small saucepan over medium heat, add the cayenne peppers, vinegar, garlic powder, salt, and pepper. Bring to a boil, then reduce the heat to medium-low.

2. Simmer for 20 minutes.

3. Remove the saucepan from heat, pour the mixture into a blender, and puree.

4. Transfer the liquid back to the saucepan, add the butter, and simmer for about 15 minutes, or until thick and smooth.

TIP: A store-bought low-sodium sauce is a great time-saving alternative.

TIP: For a lower-heat option, jalapeños (without the seeds) can easily be substituted for the cayenne peppers in this recipe.

Per serving (¼ cup): Calories: 50; Protein: 1g; Total fat: 3g; Saturated fat: 2g; Total carbohydrates: 4g; Fiber: 0.5g; Cholesterol: 8mg; Phosphorus: 21mg; Potassium: 113mg; Sodium: 150mg; Sugar: 1.5g

Food Tables

POTASSIUM

HIGHER-POTASSIUM LEGUMES*

Greater than 300 mg per cooked ½-cup serving

Black beans

Kidney beans

Lentils

Pinto beans

LOWER-POTASSIUM LEGUMES

Less than 300 mg per serving listed

½ cup chickpeas

¼ cup chopped peanuts

4 ounces tofu

2 tablespoons
peanut butter

HIGHER-POTASSIUM NUTS

Greater than 200 mg per ¼-cup serving

Almonds

Brazil nuts

Cashews

Pine nuts

Pistachios (shelled)

LOWER-POTASSIUM NUTS

Less than 200mg per ¼-cup serving

Macadamia nuts

Pecans

Walnuts

HIGHER-POTASSIUM SEAFOOD

Greater than 300 mg per cooked 3-ounce serving (unless otherwise specified)

4 clams

4 raw oysters

Atlantic mackerel

Salmon

Sardines

Tilapia

Trout

* These higher-potassium legumes can fit into a low-potassium diet as long as you stick to the serving size and avoid combining with higher-potassium vegetables, grains, and/or meat, poultry, or fish.

LOWER-POTASSIUM SEAFOOD

Less than 300 mg per cooked 3-ounce serving (unless otherwise specified)

Cod	Lobster	Shrimp
Crab	Scallops	Sole
Flounder	Sea bass	

HIGHER-POTASSIUM MEAT, POULTRY & EGGS

Greater than 300mg per cooked 3-ounce serving (unless otherwise specified)

Pork chop	Pork tenderloin	Steak

LOWER-POTASSIUM MEAT, POULTRY & EGGS

Less than 300mg per cooked 3-ounce serving (unless otherwise specified)

2 eggs	Chicken thigh	Turkey breast
3 egg whites	Hamburger	Veal
Chicken breast	Lamb	

HIGHER-POTASSIUM DAIRY & DAIRY-ALTERNATIVE FOODS

Greater than 300mg per serving specified

1 cup evaporated milk	1 cup whole milk	Turkey breast
1 cup low-fat milk	5-ounce container of	Veal
1 cup soy milk	low-fat, plain yogurt	

LOWER-POTASSIUM DAIRY & DAIRY-ALTERNATIVE FOODS

Less than 300mg per serving specified

1 cup almond milk	½ cup vanilla ice cream	5-ounce container
1 cup rice milk, unenriched	5 ounces almond-milk-based plain yogurt	of whole-milk, Greek yogurt
1 ounce cheese (most types)	5 ounces cottage cheese	5-ounce container of whole-milk,
½ cup chocolate ice cream	5-ounce container of low-fat, plain Greek yogurt	plain yogurt

HIGHER-POTASSIUM GRAINS & STARCHES (MG)**

Greater than 200mg per cooked 1-cup serving (unless otherwise specified)

1 boiled skinless medium sweet potato**	1 boiled skinless medium white potato**	Quinoa

LOWER-POTASSIUM GRAINS & STARCHES (MG)

Less than 200mg per cooked 1-cup serving (unless otherwise specified)

1 whole wheat English muffin	Bulgur	Spaghetti
2 medium slices rye bread	Couscous	Steel cut oats
2 medium slices whole wheat bread	Old-fashioned rolled oats	Wild rice
Brown rice	Pearled barley	Whole wheat spaghetti
	Peas	White rice
	Polenta	

LOWER-POTASSIUM FRUITS (MG)

Less than 200mg per ½ cup fresh, canned, or 1 small fruit (unless otherwise specified)

Apple	Dried apples, blueberries, cherries, or cranberries (¼ cup)	Pear
Applesauce		Pineapple
Apricot (fresh)		Plums
Berries	Fruit cup: any fruit, fruit cocktail	Tangerine or mandarin orange
Cherries	Grapes	Watermelon (1 cup)
Clementine	Lemon or lime	

HIGHER-POTASSIUM FRUITS (MG)

More than 200mg per ½ cup fresh, canned, or 1 small fruit (unless otherwise specified)

Avocado	Honeydew	Papaya
Banana	Kiwi	Peach
Dried fruit: raisins, dates, figs, apricots, bananas, peaches, pears, or prunes (¼ cup)	Nectarine	Plantain
	Orange	Pomegranate

**High-potassium root vegetables, such as potatoes, can be double boiled to reduce their potassium content. Simply peel, slice, and dice your potatoes and place in boiling water for 15 minutes. Drain, add fresh water, and cook until done.

LOWER-POTASSIUM VEGETABLES (MG)

Less than 200mg per 1 cup leafy greens or ½ cup fresh, cooked, or canned vegetables (unless otherwise specified)

Alfalfa sprouts

Asparagus

Bamboo shoots (canned)

Bean sprouts

Beets (canned)

Broccoli

Cabbage

Carrots

Cauliflower

Celery

Cucumber

Eggplant

Green or wax beans

Greens: collard, mustard, or turnip

Jicama/yam bean

Kale

Lettuce: all types

Mushrooms (raw or canned)

Okra

Onion or leek

Peas: green, sugar snap, or snow

Peppers: green, red, or yellow

Radish

Rhubarb

Spinach (raw)

Spaghetti squash

Cherry tomatoes

Turnip

Yellow summer squash

Water chestnuts (canned)

HIGHER-POTASSIUM VEGETABLES (MG)

More than 200mg per 1 cup leafy greens or ½ cup fresh, cooked, or canned vegetables (unless otherwise specified)

Acorn squash

Artichoke

Beet greens

Brussels sprouts

Butternut squash

Chard (cooked)

Chinese cabbage (cooked)

Corn (1 ear)

Edamame

Hubbard squash

Kohlrabi

Lentils

Parsnips

Potatoes

Pumpkins

Rutabaga

Spinach (cooked)

Tomatoes

Tomato sauce, tomato paste, tomato juice

Yams

Zucchini

Vegetable juice

PROTEIN

Protein-rich foods include meat, poultry, fish, eggs, milk, cheese, legumes, nuts, and grains. Fruits and vegetables contain very low amounts of protein and are therefore not included.

PROTEIN IN LEGUMES (G)

Per ½-cup serving cooked (unless otherwise specified)

¼ cup peanuts 9

2 tablespoons peanut butter 7

4 ounces silken tofu 10, not silken 15

Black beans 8

Chickpeas 7

Kidney beans 8

Lentils 9

Pinto beans 8

Soybeans 16

PROTEIN IN NUTS (G)

Per ¼-cup serving (unless otherwise specified)

Almonds 7

Brazil nuts 5

Cashews 6

Macadamia nuts 2

Pecans 3

Pine nuts 4

Pistachios 6

Walnuts 5

PROTEIN IN GRAINS & STARCHES (G)

Per 1-cup serving cooked (unless otherwise specified)

2 medium slices rye bread 5

2 medium slices whole wheat bread 9

Brown rice 6

Bulgur 6

Couscous 6

Old-fashioned rolled oats 6

Pearled barley 5

Peas 8

Polenta/grits 4

Quinoa 8

Steel-cut oats 7

White rice 4

Whole wheat English muffin 6

Whole wheat or regular spaghetti 8

Wild rice 7

PROTEIN IN SEAFOOD (G)

Per 3-ounce serving cooked (unless otherwise specified)

4 clams 12

4 raw oysters 17

Atlantic mackerel 20

Cod 17

Crab 15

Flounder 13

Lobster 16

Salmon 22

Sardines 22

Scallops 18

Sea bass 20

Shrimp 20

Sole 13

Tilapia 22

Trout 20

PROTEIN IN MEAT, POULTRY & EGGS (G)

Per 3-ounce serving cooked (unless otherwise specified)

2 eggs 13

3 egg whites 11

Chicken breast 26

Chicken thigh 24

Hamburger 22

Lamb 24

Pork chop 25

Pork tenderloin 24

Steak 25

Turkey breast 26

Veal 21

PROTEIN IN DAIRY & DAIRY-ALTERNATIVE FOODS (G)

Per 1-cup serving (unless otherwise specified)

1 cup almond milk 1

1 cup evaporated milk 17

1 cup low-fat milk 8

1 cup rice milk, unenriched 2

1 cup rice milk, unenriched 2

1 cup soy milk 8

1 cup whole milk 8

1 ounce cheese (most types) 6-8

½ cup ice cream 3

5 ounces almond-milk-based plain yogurt 6

5 ounces low-fat cottage cheese 15

5-ounce container of low-fat, plain Greek yogurt 15

5-ounce container of low-fat, plain yogurt 7

5-ounce container of whole-milk, Greek yogurt 13

5-ounce container of whole-milk, plain yogurt 5

SODIUM

HIGH-SODIUM FOODS TO LIMIT

Check food labels for actual sodium content per serving

Bacon

Baking mixes
(pancakes, desserts)

Barbecue sauce

Bouillon cubes

Bread

Buttermilk

Canned ravioli

Cold cuts, deli meat

Corned beef

Fast foods

Frozen prepared foods

Garlic salt

Ham

High-sodium cereals

Hot dogs

Ketchup

Microwave meals

Monosodium
glutamate (MSG)

Most canned foods
(unless specified
as no-salt-added
or low-sodium)

Onion salt

Potato chips

Salad dressings

Salted crackers

Sauerkraut

Sausage

Seasoning salt

Smoked fish

Soy sauce

Spam

Steak sauce

Table salt

Teriyaki sauce

Vegetable juices

LOW-SODIUM FOODS TO CHOOSE

Check food labels for actual sodium content per serving

Allspice

Black pepper

Canned food with no
added salt

Crackers, unsalted

Dill

Dry mustard

Eggs

Fresh fish

Fresh garlic

Fresh onion

Ginger

Homemade or
no-salt-added broth

Lemon juice

Low-sodium
salad dressings

Low-sodium
seasoning blends

Lower-sodium
breads and cereals
(check label)

Nuts, unsalted

Popcorn, unsalted

Pretzels, unsalted

Rosemary

Sage

Tarragon

Thyme

Vinegar, regular
or flavored

PHOSPHORUS

Phosphorus is found in protein-rich foods. Fruits and vegetables contain very low amounts of phosphorus and are therefore not included. Tables include total phosphorus and phosphorus adjusted for estimated bioavailability in descending order.

Plant Sources of Phosphorus: Low Bioavailability

*Adjusted phosphorus was calculated using an estimate of 50 percent bioavailability of phosphorus in plant sources.

PHOSPHORUS IN LEGUMES (MG)		
Per ½-cup serving cooked (unless otherwise specified)		
FOOD	**PHOSPHORUS**	**ADJUSTED PHOSPHORUS***
¼ cup peanuts	137	69
2 tablespoons peanut butter	108	54
4 ounces silken tofu	102	51
4 ounces tofu, not silken	122	61
Black beans	120	60
Chickpeas	138	69
Kidney beans	122	61
Lentils	178	89
Pinto beans	126	63
Soybeans	211	106

PHOSPHORUS IN NUTS (MG)

Per ¼-cup serving

FOOD	PHOSPHORUS	ADJUSTED PHOSPHORUS*
Almonds	156	78
Brazil nuts	241	121
Cashews	191	96
Macadamia nuts	63	32
Pecans	76	38
Pine nuts	194	97
Pistachios	151	76
Walnuts	101	51

PHOSPHORUS IN GRAINS & STARCHES (MG)

FOOD	PHOSPHORUS	ADJUSTED PHOSPHORUS*
1 cup cooked brown rice	208	104
1 cup cooked bulgur	134	67
1 cup cooked couscous	80	40
1 cup cooked old-fashioned rolled oats	172	86
1 cup cooked pearled barley	121	61
1 cup cooked polenta/grits	53	27
1 cup cooked quinoa	281	141
1 cup cooked steel-cut oats	219	110
1 cup cooked whole wheat spaghetti	178	89
1 cup cooked wild rice	135	68

ANIMAL SOURCES OF PHOSPHORUS: MEDIUM BIOAVAILABILITY

*Adjusted phosphorus was calculated using an estimate of 70 percent bioavailability of phosphorus in animal sources.

PHOSPHORUS IN SEAFOOD (MG)

Per 3-ounce serving cooked (unless otherwise specified)

FOOD	PHOSPHORUS	ADJUSTED PHOSPHORUS*
4 clams	164	115
4 raw oysters	294	206
Atlantic mackerel	236	165
Cod	117	82
Crab	199	139
Flounder	262	183
Light tuna	139	97
Lobster	157	81
Salmon	218	153
Sardines	272	190
Scallops	362	253
Sea bass	211	148
Shrimp	202	141
Sole	263	184
Tilapia	174	122
Trout	230	161

Phosphorus Cooking Tip: Research shows that preparing meats by boiling them in liquid can reduce the phosphorus content by 10 to 50 percent. This works best when the meat is sliced before cooking. Because the phosphorus is leached into the liquid, you'll need to discard the cooking liquid before serving.

PHOSPHORUS IN MEAT, POULTRY & EGGS (G)

Per 3-ounce serving cooked (unless otherwise specified)

FOOD	PHOSPHORUS	ADJUSTED PHOSPHORUS*
2 eggs	172	120
3 egg whites	15	11
Chicken breast	184	129
Chicken thigh	180	126
Hamburger	158	111
Lamb	173	121
Pork chop	189	132
Pork tenderloin	248	174
Steak	230	161
Turkey breast	196	137
Veal	190	133

PHOSPHORUS IN DAIRY FOODS (G)

Per serving size listed

FOOD	PHOSPHORUS	ADJUSTED PHOSPHORUS*
1 cup evaporated milk	460	322
1 cup low-fat milk	225	158
1 cup whole milk	205	144
1 ounce Brie	53	37
1 ounce cheese (most types)	130–180	91–126
1 ounce feta	96	67
1 ounce goat cheese	73	51
½ cup ice cream	69	48
5 ounces low-fat cottage cheese	213	149
5-ounce container of low-fat, plain Greek yogurt	141	99
5-ounce container of low-fat, plain yogurt	204	143
5-ounce container of whole-milk, Greek yogurt	191	134
5-ounce container of whole-milk, plain yogurt	135	95

PROCESSED SOURCES OF PHOSPHORUS: HIGH BIOAVAILABILITY (80–100 PERCENT)

The food industry is not required to provide the phosphorus content of processed foods. Foods with phosphorus additives represent the most bioavailable form of phosphorus in the diet. The following foods frequently contain phosphorus additives. Always check the ingredients of foods to be sure.

Bottled drinks (such as soda, flavored waters, juices)

Certain brands of nondairy creamers or half-and-half

Certain brands of nondairy milks

Fast food ("fast-fresh" food may be okay)

Frozen prepared meals

Many canned foods

Processed meats (includes all cold cuts, as well as breakfast meats such as sausage, bacon, and turkey bacon)

Processed sweet and savory snack foods (cakes, cookies, cheese-based snacks)

HIGH-FIBER CARBOHYDRATES

Fiber is found in vegetables, fruits, whole grains, nuts, and legumes.

HIGH-FIBER LEGUMES (G)

Per ½-cup serving cooked (unless otherwise specified)

Black beans 8

Chickpeas 5

Kidney beans 6

Lentils 6

Pinto beans 8

HIGH-FIBER NUTS (G)

Per ¼-cup serving

Almonds 4

Brazil nuts 3

Macadamia nuts 3

Pecans 3

Pistachios 3

HIGH-FIBER GRAINS & STARCHES (G)

Per 1 cup cooked (unless otherwise specified)

1 medium sweet
  potato 4

1 medium white potato 4

2 medium slices rye
  bread 3

2 medium slices whole
  wheat bread 4

Brown rice 3

Bulgur 6

Old-fashioned
  rolled oats 8

Peas 7

Quinoa 5

Steel-cut oats 5

Whole wheat English
  muffin 4

Whole wheat spaghetti 6

HIGH-FIBER FRUITS (G)

Per ½ cup fresh, canned, or 1 small fruit (unless otherwise specified)

¼ avocado 2

Apple 4

Blackberries 4

Blueberries 2

Mandarin orange 2

Pear 6

Raspberries 4

Strawberries 2

HIGH-FIBER VEGETABLES (G)

Per ½ cup cooked (unless otherwise specified)

1 cup raw baby spinach 1

Asparagus 2

Broccoli 3

Brussels sprouts 3

Carrots 2

Cauliflower 1

Collard greens 4

Green beans 2

Mushrooms 2

HEART-HEALTHY FATS

OILS

Avocado oil

Flaxseed oil (keep
refrigerated and do
not heat)

Hemp oil (keep
refrigerated and avoid
high heat)

Olive oil

Sesame oil

Sesame oil

Walnut oil (keep
refrigerated and avoid
high heat)

OMEGA-3 FISH

Atlantic mackerel (avoid
king mackerel due to
mercury content)

Rainbow trout

Salmon

Sardines

NUTS/NUT BUTTERS & SEEDS

Almonds and
almond butter

Brazil nuts

Cashews

Chia seeds

Flaxseed

Macadamia nuts

Peanuts and
peanut butter

Pecans

Pine nuts

Pistachios

Sunflower seeds

Walnuts

MISCELLANEOUS

Avocado

Low-sodium olives

Measurement Conversions

	US STANDARD	US STANDARD (OUNCES)	METRIC (APPROXIMATE)
VOLUME EQUIVALENTS (LIQUID)	2 tablespoons	1 fl. oz.	30 mL
	¼ cup	2 fl. oz.	60 mL
	½ cup	4 fl. oz.	120 mL
	1 cup	8 fl. oz.	240 mL
	1½ cups	12 fl. oz.	355 mL
	2 cups or 1 pint	16 fl. oz.	475 mL
	4 cups or 1 quart	32 fl. oz.	1 L
	1 gallon	128 fl. oz.	4 L
VOLUME EQUIVALENTS (DRY)	⅛ teaspoon	————	0.5 mL
	¼ teaspoon	————	1 mL
	½ teaspoon	————	2 mL
	¾ teaspoon	————	4 mL
	1 teaspoon	————	5 mL
	1 tablespoon	————	15 mL
	¼ cup	————	59 mL
	⅓ cup	————	79 mL
	½ cup	————	118 mL
	⅔ cup	————	156 mL
	¾ cup	————	177 mL
	1 cup	————	235 mL
	2 cups or 1 pint	————	475 mL
	3 cups	————	700 mL
	4 cups or 1 quart	————	1 L
	½ gallon	————	2 L
	1 gallon	————	4 L
WEIGHT EQUIVALENTS	½ ounce	————	15 g
	1 ounce	————	30 g
	2 ounces	————	60 g
	4 ounces	————	115 g
	8 ounces	————	225 g
	12 ounces	————	340 g
	16 ounces or 1 pound	————	455 g

	FAHRENHEIT (F)	CELSIUS (C) (APPROXIMATE)
OVEN TEMPERATURES	250°F	120°C
	300°F	150°C
	325°F	180°C
	375°F	190°C
	400°F	200°C
	425°F	220°C
	450°F	230°C

Resources

DaVita (Davita.com): Worldwide kidney health-care company with patient resources, recipes, nutrient analyzer, and support networks.

Kidney Community Kitchen (KidneyCommunityKitchen.ca): Information, resources, and recipes from The Kidney Foundation of Canada to help individuals manage their renal disease.

National Kidney Foundation (Kidney.org): A leading health organization dedicated to fighting kidney disease, offering patients facts and resources on kidney disease.

References

Centers for Disease Control and Prevention. Chronic Kidney Disease in the United States; 2019. Atlanta, GA: US Department of Health and Human Services, Centers for Disease Control and Prevention; 2019. Available at: CDC.gov/kidneydisease/publications -resources/2019-national-facts.html.

Davita Kidney Care, Diabetes, High Blood Pressure and Kidney Disease; 2020. Available at: Davita.com/education/kidney-disease/risk-factors/diabetes-high-blood-pressure -and-kidney-disease.

Geerligs P. D., B. J. Brabin, and A. A. Omari. "Food prepared in iron cooking pots as an intervention for reducing iron deficiency anemia in developing countries: a systematic review." *Journal of Human Nutrition and Dietetics*. August 2003,16(4):275-81. doi: 10.1046/j .1365-277x.2003.00447.x. PMID: 1285970.

National Institute of Diabetes and Digestive and Kidney Disease, Nutrition for Advanced Chronic Kidney Disease in Adults; 2014. Available at: NIDDK.NIH.gov/health -information/kidney-disease/chronic-kidney-disease-ckd/eating-nutrition/nutrition -advanced-chronic-kidney-disease-adults.

National Institute of Diabetes and Digestive and Kidney Diseases, What Is Chronic Kidney Disease?; 2017. Available at: NIDDK.NIH.gov/health-information/kidney-disease/ chronic-kidney-disease-ckd/what-is-chronic-kidney-disease

National Kidney Foundation, *Kidney Disease the Basics; 2021.* Available at: Kidney.org/news /newsroom/factsheets/KidneyDiseaseBasics.

Zemaitis, M. R., L. A. Foris, S. Katta, and K. Bashir. *Uremia,* StatPearls [Internet]; 2020. Available at: NCBI.NLM.NIH.gov/books/NBK441859.

Index

Acknowledgments

If you have been on this writing journey with me, words cannot express how thankful I am for your support, guidance, encouragement, and stomachs to taste test and enjoy these recipes. This cookbook would not have been possible without you.

About the Author

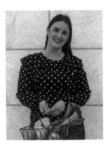

EMILY CAMPBELL, RD, CDE, MScFN, is a registered dietitian and certified diabetes educator with a master of science in foods and nutrition. With years of experience working with individuals with kidney disease and related conditions in Canada, she uses her passion for making healthy eating easy to understand, delicious, and nutritious when working with clients individually or in groups. Nutrition is complex, and Emily's goal is to break down nutrition into easy-to-understand concepts to help individuals make nutrition changes that work for their unique lifestyle and food preferences that help maintain or save kidney function.

CPSIA information can be obtained
at www.ICGtesting.com
Printed in the USA
JSHW040131041121
19984JS00006B/2